Solve Your Sleep

SOLVE *your* SLEEP

Get to the Core of Your Snore for Better Health

AMY DAYRIES,
DMD, FAIHM

MOUNT TABOR MEDIA

NEW YORK

LONDON • NASHVILLE • MELBOURNE • VANCOUVER

Solve Your Sleep

Get to the Core of Your Snore for Better Health

Published in New York, New York, by (Mount Tabor), a branded imprint of Morgan JamesPublishing in partnership with Difference Press. Morgan James is a trademark of Morgan James, LLC. www.MorganJamesPublishing.com

ISBN 9781642798340 paperback
ISBN 9781642798357 eBook
Library of Congress Control Number: 2019951055

Cover Design Concept: by:
Jennifer Stimson

Cover & Interior Design by:
Christopher Kirk
www.GFSstudio.com

Editor:
Todd Hunter

Book Coaching:
The Author Incubator

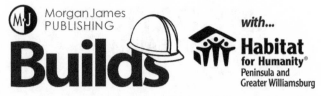

Morgan James is a proud partner of Habitat for Humanity Peninsula
and Greater Williamsburg. Partners in building since 2006.

Get involved today! Visit
MorganJamesPublishing.com/giving-back

Table of Contents

Foreword

We live in an ever-changing world. Our western model of health care can fall short at times when it comes to restoring health, for a variety of reasons, but sometimes one of those reasons can be partially attributed to rising health care costs.

Integrative Medicine involves the examination and integration of knowledge and techniques from numerous branches of health care and delivering this individualized combination to a patient in a treatment setting. I have served as the Fellowship Director in two respected Integrative Medicine Fellowship groups over the past 15 years: The Academy of Integrative Health and Medicine and the University of Arizona Fellowship in Integrative Medicine. I believe that Integrative Medicine offers an innovative approach to helping more people achieve health and wellbeing.

In this book, Dr. Amy Dayries, a former student of mine, has crafted a program that allows one to systematically move through a series of self-help and over-the-counter techniques that include herbal remedies, dietary supplements, and dietary strategies to help one achieve a better night's rest. She explores the medical research that supports about a variety of medical and dental devices currently available for the sleep-deprived individual. Amy connects the overwhelming number of health issues that can be created or worsened when one does get regular restorative sleep, and offers an integrative approach to helping people of any background and on any budget, achieve better sleep.

This book is a wonderful contribution to increasing the awareness of the many factors that affect sleep and providing individuals with a step-by-step strategy for improving their sleep and explaining when one should turn to a medical or dental practitioner for assistance. There is no question that when one experiences regular restorative sleep, one's health, energy, mood and overall wellbeing improves. Powerful medicine indeed! I highly recommend it.

Tieraona Low Dog, M.D.

June 2019

Prologue

*"Qualities you need to get through medical school and residency:
Discipline. Patience. Perseverance. A willingness to forgo sleep.
A penchant for sadomasochism. Ability to weather crises of faith
and self-confidence. Accept exhaustion as fact of life. Addiction to
caffeine a definite plus. Unfailing optimism that the end is in sight."*
– Khaled Hosseini

"Why won't my husband stop snoring, and should I be concerned?"

"My kids are telling me that I am snoring, and I am embarrassed."

These are two common complaints I often hear from my dental patients.

I am a dentist who wants to share with you how you can solve your sleep concerns. Sometimes, there are over-the-counter remedies that make a difference. Other times, a variety of techniques customized by a health provider are better for the individual.

In today's healthcare environment, patients are savvy and often know instantly when something sounds too good to be true or too much like a sales pitch. Patients and health providers alike can read research (some worthy and some that is not as credible) on the internet. When it comes to paying for information that will lead to good sleep, people are willing to pay more if the solution makes sense for the problem at hand. Since many chronic health problems of today can be traced back to an origin that involves less than optimal sleep, a variety of solutions ought to be made available so the patient can select what fits their lifestyle and budget.

Not getting good sleep has huge long-term health implications. It goes way beyond complaining about your loved one's annoying sleep habits. Being able to sort normal from abnormal conditions is critical to a healthy lifestyle. In this book, I will explore symptoms you should be aware of for yourself and others, and ways to test yourself at home to verify if you need professional help.

Dentists are often the first healthcare professional to point out to you that you may have a sleep issue because we will see evidence of tooth grinding, a scalloped tongue, or can spot a deviated septum. We dentists know that sleep can be frequently managed very well with an oral appliance.

However, sleep problems are handled in a very interesting way in today's healthcare world. First of all, only a physician can legally diagnose a sleep problem. Often, the physician's only way to treat sleep is to prescribe sleeping pills, perform surgery on a patient, or place the patient permanently on a CPAP machine to address an airway concern. However, what this paradigm is missing is that there are often natural solutions and dental completely in a gentle way. These methods have not been presented to the public under the umbrella of complete sleep solutions offerings before.

In this book, I will present all sleep paradigms: medical, natural (herbal, vitamin, and lifestyle), and the dental sleep appliances (of which there are many that address various types of sleep problems). This way, you can decide your best path or can choose to combine several methods. I will explores what good, healthy sleep looks like, and what factors may be contributing to why a person has a sleep problem. You will discover over-the-counter natural sleep remedies, connect diet and lifestyle to their potential "why" or issue, and can learn what might be a warning sign where professional help is a must. The professional help mentioned can come from several sources and is often a team approach for best results. You will learn about the protocol I use with my dental patients that has had proven results for better sleep.

Chapter 1:

Snoring Is Such a Common Problem

"Laugh and the world laughs with you, snore and you sleep alone."
– Anthony Burgess

Susan came in and slumped into the dental chair. She didn't exude her usual exuberance or smile. Susan is thirty-seven years old, a married working mother of three kids. She is really busy and goes a hundred miles an hour all the time. She is typically polished and enthusiastically sharing news about her sporty kids, her work in the IT world, or the latest with her husband. But this day was different. I exclaimed, "Wow, your energy just isn't what it usually is." She retorted, "My husband is snoring every night, and it's wrecking my sleep! I don't know how much longer I can put up with it. I'm even sleeping in the guest room occasionally just so I can better my chance of getting some decent sleep. I just don't know what to do. I've tried everything I can think of, and often my husband (Brad) thinks I'm just nagging him. I feel like I'm becoming this pestering, hysterical wife, and he doesn't want to try my suggestions." Sigh! A few years ago, I would have been less equipped to help Susan. But today, I can offer her useful advice from a variety of approaches. That's what this book is about.

In terms of suffering from poor sleep, I was there a few years ago myself. I would wake haggard after being up with my young children in the night and from hearing my husband snore. I wanted to be my on my best game at work and to be able to give my family one-hundred percent after work. This was such a challenge when sleep was not consistent or of good quality. Between juggling responsibilities as a parent, spouse, co-worker, and volunteer in the community, I easily became exhausted and generally dissatisfied with my modern life. I was sometimes told back then that I could be heard snoring. Frankly, this embarrassed me, and I was indignant that this would even be a complaint when I was already so sleep-deprived. Now I realize that had I addressed this well-meaning statement by seeking a solution, I could have felt so much more rested and less stressed. Perhaps the sadness and feeling of being overwhelmed would not have been so tough had I slept better with the time I had. At that time, I thought the trouble was how long I had to sleep, not about the quality of the sleep. My solution was to stuff earplugs into my ears before going off to bed and praying that I would not be woken up until dawn. This solution did not work so well.

As a dentist, I first encountered a situation to help someone sleep better within my own family. I knew that people in my husband's family were sort of famous snorers, which I had discovered early in my marriage on some family trips with my in-laws. My father-in-law had even been my first patient fitted for an oral sleep device because he was frequently going on scout camping trips and had been asked to move his tent away from the others in the troop due to his loud snoring. He wore a C-PAP but didn't want to bring it with him on campouts. The oral device was portable, unobtrusive, and worked well for these back-packing trips. Way back then, I realized the dental practice of the future could probably exist somewhere that only took care of sleep concerns. That was around twenty years ago, and there have been a lot of patients I have seen since then who are looking for solutions for sleep. Most patients are not back-packers but regular working people like you and me.

Even one of my young daughters began regular snoring after suffering a fall at preschool when she was four years old. Her pediatrician thought that maybe she had broken her nose, and he shrugged it off and stated that there was not going to be much in finding a solution for the nose or her snoring until she was a teenager.

As medical research has progressed over the years, physicians are beginning to fully realize the dangers of snoring because of the explosion of data that is being published regarding this topic. The key is knowledge and sharing it. Few healthcare providers are cross-trained and aware of what other types of practitioners a patient could see to solve a problem. Each branch of health providers offers their own regimen for sleep solutions. Since each profession has developed their own solution protocol, we often live in our own worlds of practice and likely do not know about the protocols of the other branches. In other words, we are trained to offer a solution within the scope of our healthcare branch for a certain problem but may not know what another type of doctor could offer for the same trouble.

As a dentist, I have been trained to make an oral appliance when I see a patient that grinds their teeth while sleeping. I may have received a lot of training on the subject of these oral appliances. I could offer either one oral appliance style for all of my patients who grind, or I may be a dentist who regularly makes eight different types of oral appliances.

There are many styles of guards, and a better dentist will understand that offering a variety of guard styles will probably best allow for selecting the most appropriate appliance for the individual, based upon the particulars of that person. A successful case will be finding a guard that both solves a problem and that a patient is willing to wear.

Egos and misunderstandings sometimes happen due to providers not appreciating how our health delivery roles may overlap and how symptoms of the patient are not contained to one body part at times. Sometimes these misunderstandings happen even between two practitioners who practice in the same field because one has more expertise in a subject than the other. The patient will have better chances of success in solving their healthcare concerns if we as a society move towards more collaboration between healthcare providers of all types. With regard to sleep, symptoms can spill over from the mouth and include the ears, nose, or throat of physician territory, for example. My wish is that this book will establish a clear understanding for the public that there are connections between systemic diseases and poor sleep and that the mouth is a place where these links may first be appreciated. I wish that the strategies and information discussed in each chapter will enable many who suffer from snoring and fatigue to find affordable solutions for their sleep, which is a critical key to reaching better health.

On a personal level, my daughter's snoring worsened in the months after her fall. My husband began to snore over time as well. I began to question why this was happening and ultimately developed a regimen that seemed to help minimize their symptoms.

In my daughter's case, I am confident that if this same traumatic fall down a staircase happened in 2019 instead of in 2006, that there would be more suggestions on the table for treatment besides waiting. In our family, we found solutions by venturing down some winding obscure paths, but these paths on the road back to health are becoming wider and better known as more people seek solutions for these sleep issues. I will address these topics a bit later so that you can navigate these paths with better understanding of the expected outcome before embarking on your journey toward caring for yourself or your loved ones.

Twenty years ago, I began to wonder more about what all this snoring meant to us all. Was snoring the inevitable way for us to be sleeping? Did it really matter? Did it have major consequences that we didn't know about?

As a healthcare provider, it behooved me to be solution-based with home healthcare. I felt I should be a living example of problem-solving health troubles. What I discovered was that the sleep issue compounded all the other health problems. In fact, what I was seeing was a "chicken or the egg" type of cause and effect. Sometimes sleep causes other health issues, and sometimes health issues worsen sleep.

I wondered, what if we could age our best? What if we could teach one another these causes and effects between sleep and health issues? What if we in the healthcare community could work together for more solution-based care instead of waiting until chronic disease sets in to treat symptoms?

Since snoring became a hot topic for me, I attended dental courses on sleep and learned about dental appliances for sleep issues. I later got involved in herbal medicine and took an eighteen-month program for health providers about how to use herbal remedies to improve all types of health concerns. Herbs were the original medicine for mankind, and some cultures have documented their uses in medicine for several thousand years. At the herbal course, I met several integrative medical doctors and learned about a two-year fellowship program in which I could enroll as a dentist. I signed up and later became the first dentist to graduate from the Academy of Integrative Health and Medicine's Inter-Professional Fellowship. My recent and ongoing endeavor is to take the knowledge I have learned through thousands of hours of study and repackage it all for the dental team. It has been an honor to share this knowledge for the last two years at the American Dental Association's National Conventions and for other academic groups as well. I also have begun a local radio broadcast called *the Whole Healing Radio Show* through the United Intentions Media Network to share unbiased current health information on a variety of topics that affect one's chances of healing and aging well.

Now I know what to say to all the people like Susan in my dental chair. I explain, "Your sleep, and his, do not have to be affected this way. If you don't address it, ultimately the marriage suffers. Snoring breaks down intimacy and health. It prevents people from getting into their restorative sleep patterns and ages you. Snoring can usually be corrected. Also, in determining why you or your loved ones snore, you can determine if there is a bigger, more serious health cause for your snoring. Imagine how well you can age and live your best life if you address this and other issues."

"Tell me more!" Susan exclaims. And that, dear reader, will be the message presented in the subsequent chapters you will see here.

Chapter 2:

The Protocol for Better Sleep Explained

"To die, to sleep – to sleep, perchance to dream – ay, there's the rub,
for in this sleep of death what dreams may come…"
– William Shakespeare, from *Hamlet*

T he purpose of this book is to present a stepwise approach to solve your snoring and sleep problems using varied options, from the simplest and least expensive treatment to the most involved and costly, so that you can sleep better starting tonight.

Using common sense, we know that for whatever reason someone doesn't sleep, it cannot be healthy long-term. Medical studies are backing this common sense. For example, we know that poor sleep quality reduces longevity from eighty years to between sixty-five and seventy years.[1]

Below some basic statistics on sleep, or rather, the lack of sleep in today's America:

- In 2016, Consumer Reports magazine published a study claiming that 27% of roughly 4,000 participants surveyed had trouble falling asleep or staying asleep most nights.
- The study cited that 68% of those surveyed struggled with sleep at least once a week. If these numbers are extrapolated across the general U.S. public, an estimated 164 million suffer from sleep loss at least once weekly.[2]
- It is estimated that 24% of adult women and 40% of adult men snore habitually.[3]
- More than 22 million Americans have something worse than snoring, in terms of a chronic insult to health, as they have actual sleep apnea.
- Studies show that 80% of moderate to severe sleep apnea is undiagnosed. In other words, the patient has no idea that they even have an official issue that can contribute to many situations of poor health over time.
- Some patients who snore have sleep apnea, which is determined by episodes where the patient stops breathing and gasps for breath. Others who have sleep apnea do not snore.
- Most patients with sleep apnea do snore.
- Snorers and sleep apniacs have many other issues such as daytime sleepiness and waking up with a dry mouth.
- Most sleep apniacs are male, overweight, and over 40 years old.[4] Children can also suffer any of these symptoms.
- Symptoms of sleep issues in children include wetting the bed, night sweats, attention deficit disorder (ADD) and attention deficit hyperactivity disorder (ADHD) types of behavior, and anxiety.[4]

- Long-term effects of not sleeping well are connected to developing diabetes, heart disease, and other chronic health issues.[4]
- There are two kinds of snoring: one that is just snoring and one that is apnea-related.

My sleep program is not a one-size-fits-all approach, but it does have steps you can start implementing at home on a shoestring budget. Not all solutions are appropriate for every reader, so we will explore contraindications and general costs for remedies suggested. If you try some of the suggestions listed in the chapters, you can share how you felt when you see your healthcare provider. This will help you and your provider select the next step on your path to wellness with more clarity.

Also, please know that my dental office trains other offices in these regimens. I will tell you where you can purchase over-the-counter remedies and will suggest at times brand names of products or devices so you know what to purchase. Some products may be unfamiliar with providers in your area, and that is okay. Often my patients have brought a new idea or product to my attention by simply mentioning it to me and inspiring me to do my own research. We are in exciting times in healthcare! I am grateful for the options we have to offer!

What follows in this book is the Core of the Snore Protocol:

1. Learn what good sleep looks like.
2. Develop herbal remedy solutions for sleep and awakeness that suit your lifestyle and personality.
3. Implement strategies to control the inflammation that makes you sick and affects sleep.
4. Understand how your vitamin and mineral levels affect sleep and how to discover your genetic makeup.
5. Discover the links between hormones and sleep.
6. Link stress and lifestyle choices to how your sleep can suffer.
7. Appreciate the medical and dental devices available on today's market that offer treatment for sleep disorders and more. Some

address symptoms, while oral appliances can address causes of poor health by remodeling the airway.

8. Integrate your individualized sleep plan using combinations of your new knowledge.

Chapter 3:

Examining How We Sleep Helps to Diagnose Sleep Issues

*"Those who dream by day are cognizant of the many things
which escape those who dream only by night."*
– Edgar Allan Poe

Most adult Americans feel best when they get at least seven hours of sleep. Many of us do not get that much time to sleep. Here are some reasons why:

- We are working longer hours (often more than sixty hours weekly at the office).

- Jobs that require participation in the global economy may create a work schedule that involves working with others who live in a different time zone.
- Shift work that many workers are doing may require work that does not fit into daytime hours.
- We often use evening hours before bedtime to entertain ourselves using screens – TV, computer, iPad – that emit blue wavelengths of light, which can disrupt our sleep by rousing our brains to some degree.
- We often also spend our evening hours managing the household since we were working during the daytime hours.

The end result for our lifestyle with regard to sleep is that we go to bed later than we should. For adults, some of the negative consequences of poor sleep over an extended period of time include:[1,2,3,4,5,6,7,19]

- Daytime sleepiness
- Difficulty focusing
- Depression
- Anxiety
- Hypertension
- Increased mortality with heart disease
- Snoring
- Sleep apnea, gasping to breathe while sleeping
- Problems in pregnancy such as gestational diabetes and pre-eclampsia
- Erectile dysfunction and/or low hormone levels
- Thyroid issues or Hashimoto's disease
- Increased rates of cancer

What about children? Kids over the age of two years need more sleep than adults, generally between eight and ten hours.

For children with poor sleep, you'll find:

- ADD

- ADHD
- Anxiety
- Asthma
- Bedwetting (enuresis)
- Dental Crowding
- Narrow dental arches/ lower face
- Mouth breathing
- Poor growth
- Swollen tonsils and adenoids
- Snoring, gasping for air

For patients who have UARS (Upper Airway Respiratory Syndrome) you will see symptoms including:

- Snoring
- Digestive symptoms
- Cold hands and feet
- Teeth grinding
- Mental fog
- Restless Sleep
- Anxiety or depression

It's now time to explore the differences between snoring, sleep apnea, and other anatomical causes of difficult nasal breathing such as having a deviated septum.

The four stages of sleep that we cycle through at night.[8]

Sleep Stages:	EEG features
Sleep stage 1: Drowsiness	Alpha dropout, vertex waves (sample of alpha dropout at arrow) ↑
Sleep stage 2: Light sleep	Spindles, vertex waves, K-complexes (sample vertex wave)
Sleep stage 3: Deep sleep	Slowing of rhythm, K-complexes, some spindles, delta activity (sample spindles)

Sleep stage 4: Very deep sleep	More slowing of rhythm, some K-complexes, delta activity
	(sample K-complexes) ↑
REM sleep:	Low- amplitude EEG, EMG flatness, with intermittent EOG activity

(sleep waves picture curtesy of https://splitrockrehab.com/memory-improvement-seniors-sleep/)

Stage 1: This lasts up to about ten minutes. When we are in light sleep, our eyes move slowly and muscle activity is slow. Our blood pressure falls and brain temperature decreases. Sometimes in this stage, we experience the feeling of falling or can have sudden but mild movements as we move into the next phase of sleep. People with irregular sleep tend to have these sudden jerky movements more often.

Stage 2: This stage lasts up to about twenty minutes. At this point, our eye movements stop, and out heart rate and brain waves slow with occasional more rapid wave bursts that can appear as sleep spindles in testing. It becomes harder to wake up someone in Stage 2 sleep. We spend most of our time in Stage 2 sleep (around 45%) as we progress from one cycle to another.

Stages 3 and 4 are slow-wave sleep, when it is difficult to wake someone.

Stage 3: Also called "Slow-Wave or Delta Sleep" This stage usually starts thirty to forty-five minutes after we fall asleep. When we progress into Stage 3, we begin to get delta brain waves (very slow brain waves) mixed with bursts of more rapid brain activity. When in Stage 3 sleep, you will often be unresponsive to noises and movements taking place near you. It is also in this phase of sleep that people will sleepwalk, have nightmares, talk in their sleep, or can wet the bed. Snoring in patients with sleep apnea is less common in Stage 3 sleep.

Stage 4: This is called REM (Rapid Eye Movement) or Paradoxical Sleep. Our first stage of REM sleep happens about ninety minutes after we go to sleep. The first stage lasts about ten minutes, and the second and typical third REM sleep stages last progressively longer before we awaken in the morning. The last cycle of REM sleep may last up to an hour. In this step, we almost exclusively produce delta waves.

During REM sleep, our breathing becomes more rapid again, and our eyes jerk rapid in various directions. Our limb muscles become somewhat paralyzed. Our heart rate increases, our blood pressure rises, and men have erections. If you awake during REM sleep, you will report having dreams. This stage of sleep is sometimes called Paradoxical Sleep because your brainwaves are active as they are when you are awake, but your body is basically paralyzed. As we age, we spend less and less time in REM sleep, whereas infants spend about half their sleep time in REM.

REM Is Important for Our Health

We should generally be getting about three courses of REM sleep nightly, and REM sleep is your restorative sleep when your body can heal. Sleep testing monitors measure REM sleep for this reason. Ideally, you would get about twenty to thirty percent of your sleep in REM. Typically the first, second, and third cycles of REM sleep get progressively longer, with the last cycle concluding shortly before you awaken for the start of the day. As we age, we get less REM sleep. When you do not get REM sleep, your body experiences increased oxidative stress and has trouble maintaining a number of variables that contribute to overall health such as maintaining body temperature. This means that the immune system is not able to function well and that you are more likely to get sick. Telomere lengths, which is a measurement associated with aging well, have been shown to be longer in patients getting good REM sleep.[17,18,19]

In our first months of life, we are already beginning to establish the sleep patterns that our bodies rely upon for growth and healing. When these patterns are irregular, there can be health implications. Infants begin forming sleep patterns in the last couple of months in utero.

They develop quiet sleep around the eighth month of pregnancy. After birth, infants sleep about sixteen hours daily, and about half of this is in REM sleep.

Non-REM in infants is slightly different from adults. There are four stages of non-REM sleep:

Stage 1: drowsiness, eyes droop, may open and close, dozing

Stage 2: light sleep, the baby moves and may startle or jump with sounds

Stage 3: deep sleep, the baby is quiet and does not move

Stage 4: very deep sleep, the baby is quiet and does not move

A baby enters Stage 1 at the beginning of the sleep cycle, then moves into Stage 2, then Stage 3, then Stage 4, then back to Stage 3, then Stage 2, then to REM. These cycles may occur several times during sleep. Babies may awaken as they pass from deep sleep to light sleep and may have difficulty going back to sleep in the first few months.[12]

Snoring Versus Sleep Apnea

Sleep apnea is a chronic sleep disorder that is denoted by a person who stops breathing while sleeping. Patients who have true sleep apnea may exhibit (but do not necessarily have all of) the following: snoring, breathlessness, daytime sleepiness, gasping for breath, waking up during sleep. Prevalence in the general population is between about two and four percent.

There are several types of sleep apnea: Central Sleep Apnea (CSA), Obstructive Sleep Apnea (OSA), or mixed type. Central Sleep Apnea occurs when the brain ceases to tell the body to breathe during sleep. It is less common than Obstructive Sleep Apnea. With Obstructive Sleep Apnea, there is a gasping for breath that occurs because there is a restriction to the airway. Sometimes your breathing is obstructed because of an anatomical issue such as a deviated septum, or it could be from a crimped section in the oral pharynx, the area of the airway located behind the teeth. Various types of scans such as a cone-beam x-ray can illuminate the details for a professional to read and show you.

Snoring occurs at different stages of sleep in those who just snore versus someone who has sleep apnea. Snoring in the regular snorer occurs mostly during Stage 3 sleep but also in Stages 1 and 2 sleep (not in Stage 4). Snoring in those with sleep apnea is less frequent in Stage 3 but is common in Stage 4 and also happens in Stage 1 and 2.

Sleep study science is called polysomnography. Tests can help explain why you snore. Also, tests explain if you have sleep issues from a sleep apnea or are just snoring. Some tests can also measure if you grind your teeth. The tests will monitor your heart rate. These days, sleep monitoring can happen at home or at a sleep center. Sleep monitoring can alert you to the types and amounts of sleep you are getting. They help your healthcare provider to identify what is going wrong. Home testing can be managed from an app for your smart phone, from a smart watch, or from a take home sleep test given to you by a professional. Professional-grade home tests costs much less than sleeping at a sleep center (several hundred dollars). Home tests also have the advantage of minimal wires and without the creep factor of someone watching you.

Below is a version of information from a take home sleep test. It depicts oxygen saturation, snoring, REM sleep, and position of the sleeper. It can be read to determine if body sleep position is correlated with a drop in oxygen saturation and snoring episodes. This test is super helpful to understand what a patient is really doing while sleeping. In this example, this patient was found to have severe sleep apnea (AHI score over 30).

There are important numbers that sleep professionals use to render a diagnosis. An app on your smart phone or FitBit will not get you these

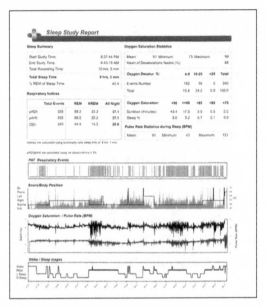

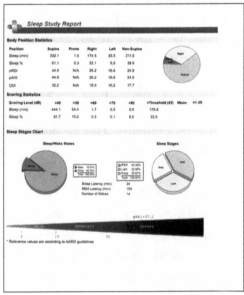

numbers, but a professional home test or sleep center test will. These numbers are measurements on which medical insurance companies base their reimbursements. They include the following:

Hypopnea is a term to describe a reduction in airflow while sleeping that is not a complete stop to breathing. It will cause a drop in oxygen saturation (which generally should always stay above 90%).

RERA is an abbreviation for Respiratory Effort Related Arousal. A patient who experiences many RERAs is often associated with a diagnosis of UARS, or upper airway respiratory syndrome. UARS indicates there may be some sort of obstruction that is making it hard for the patient to breathe.

AHI is an abbreviation for Apnea Hypopnea Index. This is the hourly average number times the person either can't breathe or when their oxygen level drops. This number is what determines the severity of a person's sleep apnea. A number over 5 is often translated to a diagnosis of a patient who has mild to moderate sleep apnea. A number over 15 is translated to indicate a patient who has a moderate to severe sleep apnea. A number over 25 indicates a patient may have a severe sleep apnea issue. A physician makes the ultimate diagnosis, although tests can be given in other places.

RDI is the number is your combined number of apnea, hypopnea, and RERAs per hour of sleep.

Your Bite Can Reflect Sleep Issues

Grinding your teeth is also associated with sleep issues. Your dentist may notice at your appointment that you show signs of wear on your teeth that correlate with grinding your teeth. Sometimes, the wear patterns do not match up to how one's teeth fit together, particularly after orthodontic work. But frequently, there is a correlation with grinding and an airway issue. Sometimes the presentation of grinding or brushing teeth at night is associated with jaw pain, and dentists call this TMJ as a reference to the temporal-mandibular joint (jaw joint). Nowadays, some sleep tests can be taken home and used to measure how much and how often you may be grinding your teeth while sleeping. These tests, particularly one by the GEMPRO company, will show if grinding episodes are happening at the end of an apnea event, which would be the body trying to compensate for the lack of oxygen. Research supports that successful diagnosis of why you may have certain nighttime activities can lead to a successful solution. In the case of teeth grinding, elimination of the airway issue can eliminate brushing teeth at night. There are dental devices that can address the airway and prevent tooth grinding while sleeping. I will cover options for dental treatment in a later chapter in this book.[7]

Restless Legs Syndrome

Restless Legs Syndrome (RLS) is a common chronic neurological disorder that is diagnosed by witnessing a patient having lots of periodic leg movements during sleep (PLMS). There is medical research that supports that most RLS patients have sleep disordered breathing. Most of these RLS patients with sleep disordered breathing actually have obstructive sleep apnea (OSA).[15]

Patients who wear a CPAP (the most popular medical device used for sleep treatment) and who still have PLMS may be having upper airway resistance that is not being solved by the CPAP. Oral appliances that we will cover later in this book (Chapter 9: Airway Size Matters) will explain how causes are addressed instead of symptoms. When you treat causes of a health issue, resolution is more complete.

There are primary and secondary forms of RLS. Three aspects of treatment should be considered for restless legs syndrome including medication (often in the form of dopaminergic drugs), lifestyle changes, and checking for and addressing potential iron deficiency. There are also known genetic components to restless legs syndrome.[9,10] Knowing this information has been part of how I got interested as a dentist in making oral sleep appliances. The dental community can affect growth in the airway that has created the upper airway resistance. While CPAP is wonderful for many sleep patients, there are a growing number of these patients who would be interested in knowing that they can address the cause of their apnea rather than just mitigate the symptoms.

Hormones in Your Body Can Influence Your Sleep

When your body's hormones are out of balance or missing, your sleep will be affected.

The pineal gland, located near the eyes in the brain, regulates our circadian rhythm so that we establish a sleep/wake cycle. It has receptors for neurotransmitters in the body for helping the body sleep called dopamine and serotonin. These help to tell your body that it is either time to make melatonin to go to sleep or that it is time to wake up. Neurotransmitters act as messengers from the brain to other tissues, and these regulate many functions and processes including sleep and general metabolism. Both dopamine and serotonin regulate similar pathways.[11,12]

Symptoms of low dopamine or serotonin can include:
- Depression or withdrawing from social situations
- Moodiness or irritability
- Cravings for carbohydrates or chocolate
- Inability to find the right sleeping position
- Insomnia
- Feelings of low self-esteem
- Anxiety or panic attacks
- TMJ (facial pain or grinding of teeth)
- Migraine headaches
- Irritable bowel syndrome (IBS)
- Obesity
- Asthma
- Addictive tendencies towards activities such as drinking alcohol, gambling, or sex (more common in men)

Dopamine

In relation to sleep, dopamine is associated with being awake. Generally speaking, dopamine acts as a sort of chemical reward system.

When you accomplish something and feel good about the situation, your brain releases dopamine. Now you feel great! For those who are not making enough dopamine, they may feel low motivation or feel like a victim, or they can experience a loss of interest in activities that used to bring joy. These people feel depressed. When your body fails to produce enough dopamine, the reason can be that you are experiencing stress, pain, or a traumatic event. Dopamine is also associated with addiction. Over time, an activity such as gambling that might have once brought an emotional high to the individual can slowly cease to bring the same amount of joy it once did. A sign of dopamine depletion could be that the individual would increase the intensity of addictive activity to obtain the same dopamine high. This is because their dopamine level is low.[11,12]

Dopamine also plays a role in digestion with relation to how your body processes insulin. It is also linked to how your body moves food through the intestinal tract, and it is a chemical that increases the mucosal lining in the intestines.

Dopamine production issues play a role in a patient who has Parkinson's disease, bipolar disorder, schizophrenia, and attention deficit hyperactivity disorder (ADHD).

Serotonin

Serotonin is the other neurotransmitter that helps regulate a metabolic pathway associated with mood. Its effect is to help you regulate your mood. Serotonin reuptake inhibitor pharmaceuticals allow your body to use the serotonin more conservatively, meaning you will get more bang for your serotonin buck, so to speak. Medical doctors often use these pharmaceuticals to help patients fight depression. Serotonin production issues play a role in those who suffer from anxiety, autism, bipolar disorder, obsessive-compulsive disorder (OCD), and social anxiety disorder.[11,12]

Ninety-five percent of your body's serotonin is found in your intestinal tract. When you eat something toxic, serotonin is the neurotransmitter released to help you expel the food quickly by stimulating contractions in the gut. Low serotonin in the gut is linked to constipation.

***

When it comes to sleep, the number of dopamine and serotonin receptors in the pineal gland of the brain influence our sleep clocks. Abnormal levels of either dopamine or serotonin can impact your ability to fall asleep, to feel awake in the daytime, or to get REM sleep. Sleep deprivation reduces the number of dopamine receptors in the pineal gland and therefore how much dopamine can be stored in the brain. This means that you can feel drowsy in the daytime because your dopamine in the brain is low. If you have a low level of serotonin, you can have a hard time falling asleep. Also, if you have abnormally high levels of serotonin in the brain tissue that have accumulated over time, you could have a hard time staying awake. High levels of accumulated serotonin in brain tissue also can reduce REM sleep.[11,12]

Dopamine and serotonin play important roles in brain/sleep function and in gut function. There are no clear ways to measure your serotonin or dopamine levels. When treating conditions, medical doctors generally prescribe for treating symptoms related to depression or sleep.

Genetic Links for Why Patients Develop These Disorders

Men and Women Sleep Differently and Have Different Sleep Disorder Symptoms!

Men and women sleep differently! Generally, women are less likely to snore or be witnessed to have apniac events where they stop breathing than men. Women also tend to have more daytime fatigue, lack of energy, sleepless nights, morning headaches, mood swings, and nightmares when surveyed in comparison to men.

Men have more episodes of complete upper airway collapse. Women have more episodes of apnea during periods of REM sleep. Women have lower AHI statistically than men, but they have longer episodes of partial airway obstruction (usually in slow wave sleep) in comparison to men.

Women who snore complain more about daytime fatigue than men. Women are more likely than men to have only partial airway obstruction and because of this have better ability to maintain carbon dioxide (needs to be at least six percent) levels in their body.

In a later chapter of this book, we will review hormonal changes that can impact women's sleep.[16]

Mouth Breathing

Mouth breathing contributes to health conditions such as asthma and overall contributes to poor sleep. Inhaling and exhaling through the mouth often creates a situation in which we pass higher than normal volumes of air through our lungs. When we mouth breathe, the additional exchange of higher than normal volume of air causes us to not hold onto at least six percent carbon dioxide in our body. The body will respond to this by clogging the nasal passages. When our nasal passages are clogged, we will breathe through our mouth with increasing regularity. Chronic mouth breathers will have changes in their oral bacteria and are at an increased risk for cavities and gum inflammation, frequently in the forms of gingivitis or periodontal disease. We will address mouth breathing more in a later chapter on lifestyle choices in this book.

Now that we know more about how we are supposed to sleep and some about associated conditions that may be caused by or can contribute to poor quality sleep, let's address some simple traditional methods to help us sleep better.

Chapter 4:

Herbal Remedies for Sleep and for Feeling Awake!

"Tired minds don't plan well. Sleep first, plan later."
– Walter Reisch

Our original medicine came from plants, and this is often referred to as herbal medicine. In some cases, plants have been documented for particular medical solutions for ailments in some cultures for over 5,000 years. Skeptics who like to cite modern "evidence-based research" sometimes argue that this traditional medicine is based on old wives' tales. It takes millions of dollars to conduct a medical research study to prove that a chemical or an herb has healing properties or can create a consistent change in the population. When an herb or plant has been known to be effective for hundreds or thousands of years, there is not much interest in the pharmaceutical industry to spend the tens of millions of dollars it would take to prove a verifiable result. Even if the money was to be spent, the result of a positive study would need to justify customers purchasing millions of dollars of crop to indirectly cover the funding of the study. Also, a pharmaceutical can be patented whereas an herb is found in nature and is not patent material. This is often why many of the herbal studies are not conducted with splashy, highly publicized modern studies. This funding is reserved for new chemicals, called pharmaceuticals, to prove delivery of consistent results when used as medicine in a population. Clinical trials are mandated before a new product is brought to the mass market of healthcare.

As a dentist, I have studied herbal remedies extensively. I have gardened for decades and have completed an herbal medicine program for healthcare providers. The origins of a number of mainstream dental products are herb-based. I am not an herbalist, but I will be explaining in this section of the book applications that herbalists use for sleep solutions. These over-the-counter products have worked for me, my family, and a number of my patients. I would consider using herbs as an excellent short-term solution for sleep issues. But I also recognize that when causes of sleep solutions are addressed, long-term solutions are more possible.

There are some studies that have been completed that do indeed show evidence of the power of herbal medicine. When possible, I will reflect these studies in my charting and writing here.

Adaptogenic Herbs

One of the major classifications of herbs is the adaptogen family. Adaptogenic herbs help the body to regain equilibrium, balance, when the body is up or down with respect to a process. The herb can have either effect on the body, and it seems to help the body better self-regulate. These herbs provide three strengths:[25]

1. Stress protection
2. Prolong the body's ability to resist stress over time
3. Increased stamina and new ability by re-establishing the body's equilibrium so that exhaustion levels are actually felt later than before.

Many of these herbs can help with sleep, nervousness, and feeling more awake. Some of the herbal remedies listed in this chapter are nerviness, meaning that they affect the nervous system.

Herbs can be taken in many forms. Some are simply ingested in food or as a garnish. Others can be enjoyed as a tea. There are companies that market herbal remedies in capsule form, and some herbs are marketed as either tinctures or essential herbs for consumption in the marketplace. Tinctures are a solution created from soaking parts of the herb in either grain alcohol or vodka, most often. Sometimes a glycerin base is used. In herbal medicine, there are traditional ratios or concentrations of plant part (specific parts are generally used for certain plants: either leaves, stem, flowers, and or root) to solvent (liquid). Herbalists label their products according to this ratio.

Essential Oils

Essential Oils are created with a chemical laboratory process called steam distillation. The distillation process of essential oil making can use vast amounts of a plant and reduce it to extreme concentrations.

When using essential oils, it is important to purchase an organic product to reduce the concentration of pesticide exposure, as any pesticide will become concentrated as the oil is created. Generally, do not use essential oils "neat," or directly, on the skin. When using essential oils on the skin, it is a good idea to dilute the oil with a carrier oil such as olive, jojoba, or fractionated coconut oil to avoid burning the skin.

Generally, my favorite herbs for inducing sleep are adaptogenic herbs. Because the herb is natural, these are generally not expensive. They also are not created specifically for a given ailment. In modern medicine, we have become accustomed to practicing a "pill for an ill" mentally. But, as you will discover in my list below, many of the herbs suggested to help aid sleep have additional uses for all kinds of healing effects.

Choose the Herb Best for You

How do you choose from a list that can have completely unfamiliar names of plants to you? Read over the description of the type of patient associate with certain herbs as a guide. There is a bit of intuition often used by the provider when selecting your herb. An herbalist can also help you in person with your choice, but if you are deciding on your own, I suggest that if there is a personality described with an herb that seems like the person you are shopping for, then that may be the best herb to try first.

If you are nervous about trying an herb, please remember that using the herb as a tea is often the gentlest way to ease into a dose. Generally, the medicinal effects of the herb are in full effect when two or three cups of tea are ingested. When purchasing an herbal tea, you want to select a high-quality tea, meaning brands that have sourced the part of the plant for the tea that contains the medicinal benefit. For example, chamomile tea is a higher quality when the flowering tops of the plant are used. When wondering, you can open the tea bag to investigate what you have. Perhaps you may consider making your own tea using bags of loose herbs you purchase or harvesting the herbs from your own garden. Refer to the resources page for suggestions on brands for ready-made teas.

Dr. Dayries' Favorite Herbal Remedies for Sleep

Ashwagandha (Withania somnifera): Ashwagandha is an adaptogenic herb in the nightshade family that has been used in Ayurvedic medicine for helping the body deal with stress. It actually lowers blood cortisol levels, can reduce inflammation throughout the body, increases mental activity, promotes better sleep, and can function as an antioxidant. The *Journal of International Society of Sports Nutrition* published a study showing that ashwagandha can help improve muscle strength, size, and recovery.[11] Other studies have demonstrated that Ashwagandha can help improve mental focus and memory. Some women from the onset of puberty through old age take ashwagandha for long periods of time. It helps improve sleep by lowering the cortisol level (a stress hormone produced and mostly dumped into the blood stream at night, around four a.m. which can rouse some from their REM sleep cycle).[12] Ashwagandha has been documented as in use for healing properties for about 5,000 years in Ayurvedic medicine. This is the nighttime herb selected for many with adrenal failure because of the cortisol effect and because it helps with thyroid issues, which often is a side effect of adrenal failure. It also helps level out women who suffer from PMS or who feel emotional turmoil. Ashwagandha is a food in some parts of the world, but here in the west, it can be found in tea or in capsule form.

An easy way to try this product is to take at night in capsule form, typically 250 mg, before bed.

California Poppy (Eschscholzia californica): This herb can be taken in capsule form to help induce sleep and relaxation as well as to prevent anxiety. I often liken this herb to the scene from "The Wizard of Oz" in which Dorothy and her fellow travelers fall asleep in a field of poppies. Traditionally, some have used California poppy as an herbal remedy for bed wetting and diseases of the bladder and the liver. It has been found to be safe to take for up to three months (the time for which it was studied).

Because the effects have not been studied yet, it is not recommended for women who are breast feeding or who are pregnant. Also, do not take when operating under the influence of other narcotics or sedatives such as benzodiazepines including Valium, Ativan, Klonopin, or Ambien, as this may cause a deeper slowing of the central nervous system that is not helpful.

A typical dose of California poppy is 100 mg/kg, but this should be checked with an herbalist or your healthcare provider for clarification for yourself. Tinctures and capsules made in combination with other herbs are available in the mass market.[10]

Cannabis: This concentration comes from hemp or its cousin marijuana. Cannabis is high in CBD Oil. It is being used for kids who have autism and ADHD. It seems to alleviate those suffering chronic pain, specifically pain from cancer. Some who have Parkinson's disease find CBD oil helps reduce tremors.[13] It reduces overall inflammation in the body. Some migraine sufferers benefit from reduction of headache pain. It acts as an anticonvulsant, sedative, analgesic, hypnotic, appetite stimulant, and has anti-anxiety effects. Medical research is showing that when used in therapeutic dosages, it has not been found to disturb any physiologic function or lead to damage of body organs. Cannabis also produces little tolerance or physical dependence.

Sales for CBD Oil are greatly increasing year after year now that legislation is legalizing growing hemp. CBD Oil contains no more than 3% THC (the hallucinogenic-inducing compound), and it can be taken to help promote sleep and reduce pain.

There is no industry set dosage recommendations for using CBD oil. Some websites on the internet recommend starting with a dosage of 25 mg.[14]

Chamomile (Matricaria chamomilla): Chamomile has been studied in babies with colic as young as six weeks old. It is a very helpful aid for colic in babies (created a 57% reduction in cholic in one study) and for general indigestion (effective in 85% of those studied to eliminate diarrhea), headaches, and for soothing anxious nerves. Chamomile is very safe; rarely do people suffer from an allergy to this herbal remedy, but there is a link between those that are allergic to chamomile and those people who have allergies to plants in the Asteraceae family.

It can easily be enjoyed as a tea, with a concentration of one table-spoon in one cup of water. A better brand of tea uses the delicate white flower tops from this plant (check for this quality by opening the bag or buying your tea loose). Some ready-made brands pair chamomile with lavender for a wonderful fragrant tea. Some herbalists believe that cham-omile can help reduce nightmares. In babies studied, a 150 mL/dose was offered no more than three times daily for a bout of cholic.[15]

When purchasing herbs for medicinal uses, I recommend choosing a brand that lists the concentrations and makeup of the tea on the labeling.

Holy Basil (Ocimum Sanctum): A different variety of basil other than what grows in your garden, Holy Basil is another adaptogenic herb that traditionally was used by yogi's to reach a meditative state. Like ash-wagandha, holy basil lowers cortisol levels. It has been shown to reduce general congestion, to improve asthma symptoms, helps with bronchi-tis. Its effect of reducing cortisol levels released into the blood stream (which impact sleep around three or four a.m.) make this herb also a great choice to try in those who have adrenal failure. Studies show it can reduce fasting blood glucose levels by seventeen percent and post-meal glucose levels by seven percent, making it helpful for an individual who is concerned about blood sugar (the diabetic or pre-diabetic patient). Holy Basil has also been found to protect the body from both heavy metal toxicity (lead, mercury, arsenic, cadmium, chromium) and the oxidative and chromosomal damage caused from radiation.[16,17]

It can be enjoyed as a savory tea, marketed as Tulsi Tea. Drinking two or three cups beginning in the late afternoon can be a wonderful way to literally (by lowering your cortisol level) reduce your stress and to lower anxiety.

Hops: This is a traditional herbal remedy that induces sleep and is found in beer. A cousin to barley and wheat, hops can be brewed into a tea. The tincture can be used to induce a deep sleep. Capsules are also available, some as low as four dollars over the counter (for sixty capsules).

Kava Kava: Translates to "talk-talk." This has been used to promote sleep, but there are concerns about hepatotoxicity (liver poisoning), so supplementing with Kava Kava regularly as a sleep aid is not recommended.

Lavender: Lavender does not taste as good as it smells, so many will combine it in a tea with chamomile for a mild sleep or relaxing aid. It can also be used as a decorative garnish for a little flavor on top of a sweet dessert. The medicinal effects of lavender relieve headaches, lower anxiety, balance hormones, lower blood sugar levels, improve sunburns, and mildly reduce cortisol production. The essential oil can be applied directly (neat form) to mosquito bites. The individual who suffers from psoriasis may find relief from pain or itching with lavender.

Many prefer or find using lavender convenient as an essential oil. Sprinkle a drop on your pillow. Another way to receive the restful benefits of lavender is to add several drops of the oil with Epsom salts (magnesium sulfate) to your bath. Lavender essential oil is the most popular oil sold for use in the United States.

Lemon Balm (Melissa Officinalis) is a popular herb in backyard gardens and is part of the mint family of plants. In ancient Greece, lemon balm was dedicated to the goddess Diana and was used for medicinal purposes some 2,000 years ago. Uses included: soothing tension, cures for skin ailments and toothaches, and a traditional help for Graves' disease (overactive thyroid because it binds to TSH – thyroid stimulating hormone – so it blocks conversion of T4 to T3). Modern day uses include using lemon balm teas to aide with PMS symptoms and menstrual cramps, and it relieves the pain and severity when ingested and applied to herpetic lesions and shingles. Steeping the leaves (approximately three teas of fresh or one tea of dried) in hot water for five minutes makes a delicious tea. This is a wonderful plant that can be used herbally for calming the kind of person who runs hard and crashes. It is safe for kids and can help settle anxiety and improve sleep. A study done at Northumbria University in England noted that students drinking lemon balm tea performed better on tests and for up to six hours later than their counterparts.[18]

Contraindications for using lemon balm regularly include hypothyroidism (underactive thyroid) and pregnancy.

Linden (Tilia cordata): This herb has been used for a variety of health benefits including insomnia, preventing epileptic seizures, reducing anxiety, and creating some cardiovascular effects. It may also have some anti-inflammatory effects and ease achy joints. It is also used to treat sinus infections, hypertension, and incontinence.[19] Linden is often enjoyed a savory tea in Ayurvedic medicine. It has mild anti-hypertensive effects (fight high blood pressure). It also has the effect of relaxing the body and therefore is a nice choice for those who have a history of the heart issues mentioned and who wish to sleep more easily. In Greek mythology, Philyra, a nymph, was turned into a linden tree by the gods after begging the gods to not leave her among mortals.

Contraindications for use: Linden tea has been traditionally used as a sedative in some cultures for infants. There has been a study published showing evidence of C.botulinum being present in three percent of loose tea samples, which suggests that there is a risk in infants studied contracting botulism from Linden tea.[20] So, the conclusion of the study is to not give infants linden tea. It is also recommended that pregnant or nursing moms not drink this tea.

Dosage: Generally, less than four grams daily.

Macuna pruriens (aka Velvet Bean, Lacuna bean, Lyon bean, Cowage): This is an African legume and is high in protein. It is a food in some parts of the world. When touched by the skin, it creates a feeling of extreme itchiness. It is used in both Unani medicine and in Ayurvedic medicine. It contains a high level of L-dopa and has been traditionally used to treat Parkinson's disease because of the L-dopa content. It also contains trace amounts of serotonin, nicotine, and bufotenine. It also has anti-diabetic effects and contains anti-oxidants.[7,8] It is sold over the counter as a liquid supplement or as a capsule in the United States. Taking this as an herbal medicine has been found to improve sleep quality in both men and women who took this supplement every night for one month. It stimulates growth hormone release. Sleep quality was measured by how long it took to fall asleep, how long the subject slept, length of sleep, sleep disturbances, and daytime sleepiness. No contraindications were found in this study.[9]

Motherwort (Leonurus Cardiaca): The aerial (upper) parts of this plant, a member of the mint family, are used for herbal medicine. Its traditional uses include managing:

- Emotions (for someone in grief)
- Premenstrual cramps, amenorrhea or dysmenorrhea, PMS symptoms
- Mild effects on lowering blood pressure.
- Treating someone in pain from shingles and herpes simplex
- For the individual who suffers both anxiety and hypertension, motherwort has been medically proven to ease these symptoms and to improve sleep.

It has also been used for those suffering from hyperthyroidism, atrial fibrillation, or endocarditis. In one study, motherwort was found to be significantly helpful for reducing symptoms of anxiety and depression in 32% of patients studied and had a moderate effect on 48% of those studied.[22]

Using motherwort is contraindicated in those who are pregnant because it can induce uterine spasms and cause nausea.

A typical dose is 100-200 mg before bedtime, but the dose can be up to 500 for sleep and anxiety.

Passionflower (Passiflora): Monks traditionally took this herb when they felt overwhelmed, compassion fatigue from helping others, or even for the effects of emotional depression. It has been linked to help with feelings of anxiety, ADHD, cardiac rhythm abnormalities, and symptoms of menopause in numerous places. It was marketed in a number of over the counter herbal sleep remedies until the FDA banned this marketing practice in 1978 citing lack of proven effectiveness. It has been proven to help with symptoms of depression without impairing motor or memory skills.[21] It is often enjoyed as a tea but can also be purchased as a capsule.

Generally, drinking two to three cups daily helps with managing emotions and therefore helps the individual be able to ease into sleep.

Skullcap (Scutellaria lateriflora): Skullcap is a cousin to spearmint and is a Native American plant. The leaves and stems are used as a tea or tincture to reduce anxiety, stress, and insomnia. Skullcap has been medically studied and shown to greatly reduce anxiety and improve mood without adversely affecting mental cognition.[23] Skullcap is a good choice when the patient is the type of person who wakes up in the middle of the night ruminating about the stressors in their life. When one ingests skullcap, it is like someone has indeed placed some sort of cap upon one's brain that will take away the worries of the day. Skullcap does also reduce blood pressure slightly. Take it just before bedtime. This is also available as a capsule.

It is not recommended for pregnant or breastfeeding women. Some varieties of skullcap can interfere with cyclosporine drugs, which are often used for transplant patients to prevent rejection of the transplanted organ. Also, skullcap should be used with caution in a person with low blood pressure, as it can cause a slight drop in blood pressure.

Dose is typically one to two grams of dried herb or one dropperful of tincture.

Valerian (Valeriana officinalis): The root of the plant is used in herbal medicine. This is a potent sleep-inducing sedative.[24] It has been used for patients with restless leg syndrome. The person taking valerian may awake with lethargy but will sleep soundly. This is available as a tea, tincture, or capsule over the counter.

Do not mix with barbiturates or alcohol.

A typical dose of valerian is 300-600 mg of the rhizome, thirty minutes to two hours before bedtime. If taking as a tea, make a solution containing two to three grams of dried valerian root per cup of water, allowing it to steep for about ten to fifteen minutes.

Additional Supplements That Also Help with Sleep

Melatonin: Melatonin is used to help induce sleep, and it is most effective when taken several hours before bedtime. Our bodies make melatonin naturally from exposure to sunlight. Melatonin functions to help the brain with regular circadian rhythm. Melatonin supplementation has also been used to help alleviate symptoms in those who suffer from autoimmune conditions.[1,2] Melatonin supplies will be depleted by the drugs alprazolam (Xanax) and diazepam (Valium). Vistaril, an antidepressant, is also linked to melatonin depletion. Melatonin can also be depleted by beta-blocker pharmaceuticals.[13]

5-HTP: This is a precursor for melatonin and can be taken just before going to sleep to prevent nighttime arousals. If you wake up for a necessary event, such as a fire alarm, a young child with needs in the night, or because you really have to use the bathroom, you will still generally be able to go back to sleep if you take 5-HTP before bedtime. There is cause for concern about taking 5-HTP for a long period of time. There are some concerns that have been voiced about how the body will react if 5-HTP has been taken for many years on a regular basis because it can deplete the balance of serotonin and dopamine stores in the body by cancelling out some of your body's natural regulatory processes that are measuring production of these chemicals.[3]

For temporary sleep improvement when you are not taking an anti-depressant, 5-HTP capsules may help you.

Dr. Dayries' Favorite List of Adaptogenic Herbs for Awake-ness:

See the Tables section of this book for details on suggested dosing and for contraindications.

Why discuss herbs for feeling awake when your problem is snoring and sleeping? As you read further, you will discover that hormones greatly affect your sleep because of their influence on organs such as the adrenal glands and thyroid. Balancing the thyroid and adrenal glands during the day with herbs will assist your nighttime efforts.

Eleuthero / Siberian Ginseng (Eleutherococcus senticosus): Eleuthero is also called Siberian Ginseng. It is a specific variety of ginseng and is great choice for someone who is beginning to struggle with the pressures of daily life and who is unable to reduce this stress load presently. In the elderly, eleuthero has been studied and shown to improve feelings of mental health and ability to be social.[27]

People who should avoid eleuthero or use it with caution include those with hypertension, those pregnant and nursing, those with sleep apnea, and in those taking digoxin or hexobarbital.

If you are taking too much, you may experience anxiety, insomnia, confusion, or irritability.

This herb can be purchased ground up or in capsule form. Its mild taste allows for it to be added as a garnish over salads (use one teaspoon) or in smoothies when used in ground form. Typical dose ranges from 300-1200 mg/day.

Maca: This herb is helpful for those who need to reboot their libido. It can be commonly found as a savory, spicy tea. It traditionally has been used to increase sex drive. It does have hypertensive effects, so someone who has high blood pressure should perhaps try another herb for added pep in their life.[28]

Rhodiola (Rhodiola rosea): This flowering herb is used for those suffering with autoimmune issues or for those who need a stronger pickme-up than eleuthero. Rhodiola has also been studied for its anti-depressive effects. While one study found rhodiola to be not as effective for treating depressive symptoms as sertraline (Zoloft), rhodiola did improve the symptoms without the adverse side effects of the pharmaceutical. Some of the patients on sertraline in the study had to discontinue use of the pharmaceutical due to heart palpitations, headaches, insomnia, and sexual dysfunction. No one had to discontinue the use of rhodiola in the study.[25,26] Rhodiola can promote effects that have been likened to drinking a super-size energy drink but without the jitters one can have with a caffeine buzz. Traditionally, the Vikings ingested this herb, and its properties were attributed to the fortitude exemplified by the Vikings in battle. It can be found over the counter in either tincture, capsule, or powder form.

Traditionally, it is used for those who are chronically exhausted, who feel burned out from life's responsibilities. It helps decrease fatigue and can improve symptoms of depression and been studied for its ability to ease symptoms of fibromyalgia.

Contraindications for using rhodiola are not known.

Dosage is typically about 250 -700 mg/day, typically split into one or two doses.

Saint John's Wort: This herb has been proven to be as effective as antidepressants when used for longer than three months' time. It has been studied and found to be helpful in those who feel depressed from Seasonal Affective Disorder (SAD) and in those who suffer from fear or anxiety. It eases the emotions of fear, anxiety. It has been studied for those who have anorexia. Results are usually noticed after two weeks of regular use. St. John's Wort has been shown to upregulate the pathway referred in medicine as PXR receptor in the intestines. This means this herb could affect de-enhance how Vitamin D is used.[4]

This herb is used as a fresh strength extract, enjoyed as a tea (two to three cups dosage) or ingested as a capsule (1350 mg extract, 2.7 mg hypercins).

Do not take St. John's Wort with SAMe or other anti-depressants because this can lead to psychotic episodes from a buildup of serotonin. This is called serotonin syndrome.

Schisandra (Schisandra chinensis): This adaptogenic herb is also referred to as five-flavored fruit in Traditional Chinese Medicine (TCM) and is called Wu Wei Zi. Different parts of the fruit provide stimulation for all five flavors: sweet, salty, pungent, sour, and bitter. This fruit was used by the Soviets in World War II when they noted that in TCM schisandra was used by hunters to reduce thirst, as a nerve tonic (provide relaxation), to reduce hunger and exhaustion, and to improve night vision.[25] This herb has also been noted to ease hot flashes and heart palpitations in menopause.[30] It is a free radical scavenger and may help detox from heavy metals or act as an antimicrobial.[31]

Contraindications: Schisandra induces phase 1 drug metabolism and competitively inhibits phase II detoxification. In pharmaceuticals that are metabolized by the cytochrome p-450 pathway in the liver, please check with your doctor before trying this over-the-counter herbal remedy. Also, do not use in pregnancy as this herb has been used in high doses to stimulate labor.[31]

Dose: One or two 200 mg capsules when used in supplement form. The berries traditionally eaten can be purchased from some Asian grocery stores.

Shatavari (Asparagus racemosus): This herb has been used for women seeking more libido and energy. It translates to "she who has a hundred husbands" or "she who is acceptable to many." It has mild energy-promoting effects and has been used in women from puberty through old age, especially during menopause. It supports mild production in a nursing mother. Despite being used for thousands of years in Ayurvedic medicine, how it works is not well understood. It is commonly used to help with female reproductive issues that are affected by stress. Stress creates reactive oxygen species, which contribute to inflammation and imbalances in multiple metabolic systems. It has actions on the ovary, and we need more studies to fully understand how this works. What we do accept in the herbal medicine world is that shatavari seems to help rebalance female hormones, improves symptoms related to polycystic ovary syndrome (PCOS), helps with normal follicular growth and development, oocyte quality, and improves overall fertility by reducing the effects of stress and reducing the creation of reactive oxygen species in the body.[29]

Contraindications: This herb should not be used by anyone who is allergic to asparagus. No significant adverse effects are noted with shatavari.

Dose: When used as ground powder, about a quarter to a half teaspoon is appropriate and tasty in a smoothie, in a glass of warm milk, in ghee, or in honey. The powder is a convenient way to use shatavari, but some can purchase shatavari as a capsule.

What brands of over the counter products do I recommend?

I search for products that are organically grown, preferably in the U.S.A. Some grocery store chains carry herbal products, but an herbal store will usually give you a wider variety of choices and will employ a salesforce that will be able to answer specifics about their inventory. I prefer if I can determine where and by whom the herb was grown. It is also preferable to buy sustainably produced agriculture.

About Caffeine

Caffeine is the active ingredient that promotes the popularity of many beverages on the market increases alertness such as coffee, tea, cola, and cocoa. In a study of caffeine's implication for alertness in athletes, it stimulates the central nervous system, autonomic nervous system, cardiovascular, respiratory system, and kidneys. When taken before exercise, it increases endurance and ability in high-intensity exercise.[5,6] On a typical day, eighty-five percent of Americans use caffeinated products, and the average daily consumption is 300 mg. A dose of about 500-600 mg will affect you like a dose of amphetamine drug (speed). While the typical American dose is about three times more caffeine than the daily average throughout most of the world, English and Swedish citizens average double the daily American average through tea consumption. Caffeine begins to kick into our system to promote alertness about thirty minutes after oral consumption. When caffeine is consumed daily, there is a tolerance established by the body, and it is less effective as a stimulant.[7]

Sleep is affected by caffeine consumption. Caffeine makes it harder to fall asleep and can make your total sleep time shorter than it would be without its presence in your body. Caffeine can also reduce the amount of Stage 3 and Stage 4 sleep you need. One study found that caffeine consumption within six hours of bedtime reduced total sleep time by one hour. These effects can be magnified in the elderly. Caffeine consumption should be monitored in pregnancy, as it can cause complications by acting as a diuretic (creating a dehydrated state). It is recommended that you do not drink more than 300-400 mg/day (about three or four cups of coffee). A typical cup of black tea or most twelve-ounce sodas contains 55 mg of caffeine, whereas a typical cup of coffee contains about 95 mg. Vivarin contains 200 mg of caffeine. Decaffeinated coffee contains less caffeine (from less than one percent to less than half of regular coffee, depending on brewing method and brand) than regular coffee but should still be eliminated from the diet within six hours of sleep.[7]

A Note About Sleeping Pills

It has been demonstrated that many prescribed sleeping pills by their doctors are not actually suffering from less than seven hours of sleep. Sleeping pills have been shown to increase sleep times to be excessively longer than normal. There is also a statistically significant mortality rate in those taking sleeping pills. Therefore, there are risks in taking hyponotic drugs for the long term. There may actually be greater mortality risks from taking sleeping pills and abnormally long sleeps associated with their use than with risks of short sleep or insomnia.[32]

On a personal level, part of the inspiration to write this book is because of two patients of mine. One of these patients is a very dear friend who became fearful of trying to sleep without taking a sleeping pill. She took sleeping pills for almost ten years. Her blood pressure crept up, and her alcohol use was regular due to taking executives out for sales meetings. Her long-term health was a great concern of mine. At the time in her life when she became hooked on sleeping pills, she had an excessively high-stress job and had suffered a great loss in her family. Another patient of mine sleepwalked under the influence of a commonly prescribed sleeping pill. He ended up falling down a flight of stairs and broke his lower jaw into two.

With all of my heart, I wish for my patients and loved ones to find sleep solutions that are supportive of their health and overall wellbeing.

Herbs are our natural source of medicine. They are generally gentle and address a number of issues simultaneously for a short while.

Case Study: Julie, the Business Owner Who Can't Sleep

Julie is a business owner who can't sleep because she is worried about her teenage kids staying on track. She also runs her own small business with some of her neighbors. She has had some upcoming events to showcase her artwork at a local market that sells to businesses all over the southeast. Julie's husband travels for his work, and he is frequently out of town during the week. This means Julie is basically a single mom with the kids during the week.

Her business took off last year when it was featured in a fashion magazine. This is why she has hired some of her neighbors to help grow what was previously a fledgling start up being run out of her basement. She is super excited that people are loving her work and she so desires to meet rising demands with all the new orders for her artwork that are pouring in via internet sales. She is waking up thinking about how to manage the new growth and feels so stressed out.

She sometimes also has personal troubles not appearing to have favorites amongst her growing work team. Once she wakes up (which first starts around three a.m.), she can't get back to a deep sleep and sometimes suffers hot flashes at night. She has tried going to bed sooner in the evening, but her kids' loud music often makes this difficult. She is often extremely tired in the daytime now but cannot rest because of the expansion in the business. She is drinking a whole pot of coffee or other super caffeinated drinks to make it to the end of the day with her eyes barely open.

Julie came in for a dental visit with me and relayed her troubles. She had more gingivitis (gum inflammation) than usual, and she was grinding her teeth more (as evidenced by her newly chipped back tooth). My suggested solution for Julie was:

1. Continue to work on establishing a sleep routine. This means eliminating blue screen lights (end work at least two hours prior to sleep whenever possible and also eliminate TV or dim your phone light. This is covered in a later chapter on Stress and Lifestyle).

2. Try 400 mg magnesium citrate before bed to relax muscles. Taking an Epsom salts bath (magnesium sulfate) can be helpful with a few drops of lavender essential oil added to the bath water.

3. I suggested Julie take a probiotic several times a week to help with gum inflammation and to fortify her immune system with bacteria that her body needs most.

4. Drink two to three cups of passionflower tea in the late afternoon to ease stress, relax more, and to temper the concerns of offending others at work.

5. Take a 5-HTP before bed since she is waking in the middle of the night. If Julie was having trouble falling asleep, then melatonin might have been a better option. Julie might also take a capsule of 200 mg schisandra before bed to ease hot flashes.

6. If she is tired in the day, Julie can try sprinkling a teaspoon of ground eleuthero powder into her breakfast (a smoothie) to increase her energy.

7. I asked Julie to limit her coffee to two cups daily.

Julie emailed me about a month after her appointment to report that she was sleeping much better and that her big orders were being met! All was well! She thanked me for the suggestions!

Julie returned for a six-month checkup and no longer had gum inflammation. Her stress was not so much an issue. She reported not needing the 5-HTP much anymore but planned to keep a stock of it around for an emergency, I-have-to-get-a great-night's-rest-tonight situation.

Case Study: Snoring Holly with Sjogren's Syndrome

Sjogren's syndrome is an autoimmune disease which affects about seven million people in the United States, mostly women over the age of forty. It is an autoimmune condition with symptoms including dry eyes and mouth. Often patients with Sjogren's also have damage to kidneys, with lung function, liver detoxification issues, and thyroid issues. Many of these patients also suffer from fatigue and arthritis-like pain. In fact, about half the time a patient has Sjogren's, there will also be another autoimmune condition at hand such as arthritis, Hashimoto's, lupus, Raynaud's disease, or scleroderma. A physician with a blood test confirms the diagnosis.

Patients with Sjogren's often have burning mouth syndrome, gum inflammation, tooth decay, mouth sores, loss of normal taste, swollen salivary glands, dry cough, dry lips, difficulty swallowing, heartburn or

GERD, and joint pain. They also often have vaginal dryness, chronic fatigue, muscle pain, and weakness and skin rashes. They are also at a higher risk than the average population for lymphoma.

Holly, a forty-three-year-old mother of a toddler came in to see me for a routine hygiene visit. She had always been an exercise maniac. She has a home gym and is very disciplined about diet and lifestyle. She has a high-profile job with a corporation in my area that has twenty-one offices. Holly had lost some weight since her last visit and complained about her low energy and daytime fatigue. She had been diagnosed with Sjogren's syndrome about two months earlier after repeatedly seeing her doctor with symptoms of fatigue. The doctor's suggested solution to treat Holly's Sjogren's symptoms was to take a series of eye drops and some medicines for cancer that were very expensive which Holly found made her feel bad. Holly's mouth had some signs of Sjogren's including dryness, a small new cavity at the gum line on two of her back teeth, and redness everywhere from a yeast infection (oral candidal infection). When asked, Holly reported that her vitamin D levels tested around 28 ng/mL (low). Holly is not sleeping well and has worn an orthodontic retainer to prevent her teeth from moving. She had popped a veneer off of one of her front teeth recently, which is often an indication of grinding teeth while sleeping, a sign of an underlying sleep issue. She had previously worn a nightguard but had stopped because her husband said it seemed to make her snoring worse.

She asked me if there was anything else she could do to treat her Sjogren's and feel better. I asked her to check with her doctor about everything we discussed so that she could ensure that all her medical routines were known to all of her providers.

Holly was placed on the following suggested regimen:

1. Anti-inflammatory diet
2. Fish oil, 3000 mg per day, high-quality, higher in EPA to DHA fatty acids. Fish oil high in EPA has more anti-inflammatory

effects than other types of fish oil. With autoimmune conditions, inflammatory cell counts are generally higher and white blood cells are attacking normal cells. We want to counter this activity by lowering the body's response to inflammation. This may help reduce Holly's joint soreness and feel better overall.

3. Borage oil or flax seed oil to support moisturizing tissues

4. A solution of fractionated coconut oil (one tablespoon) mixed with two drops of cinnamon oil to alleviate oral candidiasis (thrush). The oil is moisturizing, and the cinnamon is highly effective for fighting the yeast infection.

5. We recommended eliminating drinks that are diuretic and acid-creating in the mouth. This includes drinks that contribute to dehydration including coffee, sodas, and tea.

6. Liposomal vitamin C supplements, 1000 mg daily to help with general healing.

7. Vitamin D supplement, 5000 mg daily with the agreement with Holly that she get her vitamin D levels tested within the next three months to ensure we get her levels over 70 ng/mL.

8. Holly took with here our take-home sleep test. Results supported that she has an AHI Score of 7.5, suggesting at least a mild sleep issue. Significant snoring was reported on the study. We decided in the short run to make Holly a snoreguard to stop the grinding of teeth and reduce snoring. She will retest with a sleep study in six months to determine if getting her vitamin D levels higher and her life in better order with using her small mouth guard at night is enough to support her health.

Chapter 5:

Inflammation and Exercise: Their Role in Sleep

"I treat myself pretty good. I take lots of vacations, I eat well,
I take supplements, I do mercury detox, I get plenty of eater
and I stay away from drama and stress."
– Reba McEntire

The Connection Between Health and Sleep

One of the most important topics to understand is connecting poor sleep with inflammation and chronic disease. Poor sleep is connected to heart disease, diabetes, osteoporosis, Alzheimer's disease, Parkinson's disease, and obesity.

47

As a dentist, I see overall health through oral examinations. About ninety percent of the time when there is systemic disease, there will be a sign of this disease in the mouth. Parts of the body are all connected by the same blood supply and are all housed within the same skin. When there is good oral health, generally there is good overall health in the patient.

Oral Health = Overall Health

My dental assistant, Carol, told me once that it used to be said in the South that it was a good idea to check out a person's teeth before considering marriage! At the time, it was a funny thought, but now knowing how oral health affects overall health and is related to systemic health, the legend makes for good common sense.

Most systemic disease (disease affecting the whole body) has visible signs in the mouth, and most of the body's immune system cells are located in the gastrointestinal tract. So, keeping the gut in its best health ends up being a golden ticket to overall health, including improving sleep. Imagine how if you are suffering from gut issues, you may be more likely to get up in the night to use the bathroom. Twenty percent of Americans are actively having gut troubles, and it's very likely that it's part of the reason they are not sleeping as well as they could.

Let's examine why gut health can worsen and solutions for this trouble.

Gut health and oral health are one and about the same.

Oral Health = Overall Health and Good Sleep

The bacteria in digestive system (which starts with the mouth and goes all the way to your anus) influence how your body functions on all levels. They influence how you digest food (contribute to development of leaky gut and irritable bowel syndrome (IBS)), how you feel (influence depression), and indirectly how your brain functions (how you sleep).

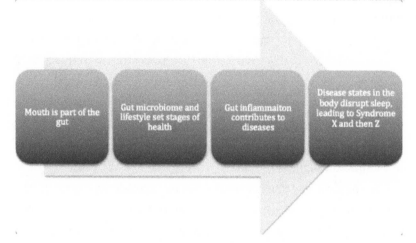

More specifically, only certain types of bacteria cause cavities in teeth and gum disease (periodontitis).

We have lived in a medical paradigm that has called for eradication of bacteria! In other words, when someone has an infection that is caused from bacteria, our go-to for treatment for the last seventy-five years has been to take an antibiotic, indiscriminately destroying good and bad bacteria.

Other chemical exposures can alter the gut bacteria. This includes frequent usage of ibuprofen, sugar, alcoholic beverages, and acidic foods (such as canned foods). There is also evidence that chemicals used in agriculture can alter the bacteria in your gut such as glyphosate (an herbicide – to learn more about glyphosate and its connection to chronic illness and sleep, see Figure 1 later in this chapter).

The issue is that some bacteria will be living inside us as soon as our antibiotics are done, the alcoholic beverage is drunk, the pill has been metabolized. The bacteria that are fed best thrive the most. When the body becomes a more acidic environment through sugar consumption and acidic foods, the bacterial population changes. Generally, speaking, most bacteria living inside us are potentially killed during antibiotic therapy. After conclusion of antibiotic therapy, there will be a race to repopulate the human. Whichever repopulates first will have significant portions of real estate and will dictate function inside your body. Due to mass usage of antibiotics across the human race for the last few decades, the bacteria have developed resistance to our antibiotic onslaught in recent years because they have genetically morphed into being able to live through the onslaught. These beings are more simply structured than the human and take fewer generations to morph than we do. We have not yet formulated new antibiotics to keep up with the treatment paradigm of unleashing antibiotics to seemingly restore health in the body.

So, over the last number of decades, the numbers and types of bacteria in our guts have changed. Also, when you snore or mouth breathe, you will change the bacteria in your mouth. We do not carry numbers of the same strains of bacteria as we used to as a populace. Thus, we are seeing vast numbers of people develop other diseases, particularly auto-immune diseases and digestive problems that cascade into other troubles. Indirectly, sleep can become a symptom or a contributing factor of these gut changes: the chicken or the egg analogy. There is also something called the Old Friends Hypothesis by Charles Raison M.D., Graham Rook M.D. and Christopher Lowry M.D. "Ancient commensal bacteria, parasites, and virus that induce tolerance and peacekeeping in micro-biomes of body are being tampered with due to modern hygiene, urbanization, antibiotic use, pesticides... devastate gut biome health, increasing rates of disease."[1]

There is a term used in healthcare today called Metabolic Syndrome (or Syndrome X), and it often develops when the microbiome of the gut has been altered. This term used in the medical profession describes if you have a sedentary lifestyle and three of the following:

- Abdominal obesity (waist size over 40 inches in men; over 35 inches in women)
- Elevated Blood Fats (triglycerides greater than 150 mg/ dl)
- Low HDL (aka cholesterol levels less than 40 mg/dl men, less than 50 mg/dl women)

- Elevated blood pressure (over 130/85)
- Elevated fasting blood sugar (over 100 mg/dl)

What we know is that people who have developed Metabolic Syndrome often are suffering from poor sleep and that prevalence of metabolic syndrome happens forty percent more often in those who have sleep apnea.[2] When metabolic syndrome is paired with sleep apnea, the medical profession calls it Syndrome Z. As a dentist, I noticed that people with metabolic syndrome often have gum inflammation.

So, poor sleepers are much more likely to have increased inflammation (including gum infections). They often eat diet that is nutrient poor, and commonly, they do not engage in regular exercise programs. The increased inflammation predisposes people to heart disease, diabetes, and kidney disease.

Also, there are some internal body chemical changes that occur with Syndrome X and Z. These include the chemicals called: C-reactive proteins (CRP's) and Interleukin 6 (Il-6). When you develop Metabolic Syndrome, you end up with serum levels of plasma IL-6 and CRP concentrations that have been determined to predict adult depression eleven years after being traced in the blood stream. There was a scientific study conducted between 1991-1993 and followed up on in 2002-2004 conducted in Britain called the Whitehall II Study which found that increased levels IL-6 and CRP concentrations adults could be used to predict depression in adults, whereas typical reasons or history of depression could not predict an increase in inflammation. So, it has been concluded that inflammation precedes depression when it comes to people having fatigue and feelings of hopelessness and sadness, loss of life-drive that comes with depression. IBS, gingivitis, tobacco use, depression, CVD, acute infection, and PTSD can develop in relation to poor sleep and metabolic syndrome.[1,2,3]

To prevent Syndrome X or Z, it is best to know your blood sugar levels, triglycerides, and cholesterol levels.

When considering cholesterol as a health factor, you may have heard references to the terms LDL and HDL. LDL is an abbreviation for lower density lipoproteins, and HDL is an abbreviation for heavy density lipoproteins. Both of these circulate in our bloodstream. They have different roles in our health state.

In a nutshell, too much LDL is associated with the conditions of inflammation including hypertension and cardiovascular disease conditions. LDL can cause fatty deposits on the walls of blood vessels, leading to risk of stroke, heart attack, and atherosclerosis. Some have simplified the cholesterol factor in health by tagging LDL as "bad cholesterol." HDL functions as a sort of garbage truck to clean up toxins and an overload of LDL particles in the blood stream so that these can be excreted eventually. HDL has been tagged as "good cholesterol" sometimes. You will have both LDL and HDL no matter what your state of health or inflammation is.

Too much of either spells a recipe of an inflammatory state. Physicians have tested HDL and LDL levels for years, but we are finding out that there may be some other numbers that are as useful or even more reliable as a predictor of inflammation and cardiovascular disease. Also a particle size test, which breaks down in lab results the percentages that exist of cholesterol particles in their various sizes, is probably a better overall predictor of true risk than just knowing LDL and HDL numbers. Apo-B is another one of these numbers that may prove to be more useful over time for identifying inflammation and cardiac risk.

Apo B is an abbreviation for Apolipoprotein B-100. It is another marker physicians use to determine your potential for disease states or predict risks associated in an absence of health. Apo-B is a protein that is involved in the metabolism of lipids.[4] Elevated numbers of Apo B correspond to elevated levels of LDL and more cholesterol that is not HDL type. Sometimes Apo B is attributed to a genetic marker identified by blood testing at your doctor's office. Populations that have higher levels of Apo B include people who are diabetics, suffer from hypothyroid, kidney disease, and those who are pregnant. Apo B numbers can be decreased when lifestyle choices are made such as reducing weight through diet and exercise.[5]

Realize that ratios matter (LDL vs. HDL), eat well, and exercise! All those science numbers are found in routine blood testing from your doctor. Snoring is correlated to changes in the ratios of LDL to HDL and higher levels of Apo B.

Heavy Metal Loads

Heavy metal burdens are what your body has been exposed to over the course of your lifetime. In the world of modern integrative medicine, heavy metals are closely linked to a number of inflammatory disease conditions. You can be exposed to heavy metals even before you are born if your mother has a toxic load. Exposure also can happen through a variety of sources including ingestion of contaminated food or water sources, handling chemicals, and amalgam dental fillings. Most recently, the municipal water supply in Flint, Michigan became the subject of a national news story due to the lead contamination of the tap water due to delivery through pipes that leached lead into the water.

The eleven heavy metals that patients are commonly tested for are arsenic, cesium, gallium, mercury, lead, cadmium, thallium, copper, tin, aluminum, and zinc. You can get tested for heavy metals either by blood, urine, or hair testing. Blood tests will only show exposure for the last 48 hours. Heavy metals are either absorbed into tissue or excreted after this time. Your heavy metal load is generally better reflected in either hair or urine test. There are arguments between practitioners about which is the better or safer way – hair or urine – to test their patients' heavy metals. Some practitioners have given heavy metal tests in the past by dosing a patient with a chemical surfactant such as DMSA or others. Some feel that this way of testing can pull the toxic metal out of tissue where it can then be redistributed among tissue before excretion. Hair testing does not require this surfactant spiking method.

Heavy metals bind to hormones and enzymes easily, which can reduce a patient's ability to detox or make enough chemicals for required metabolic processes such as good digestion or the ability to release hormones that regulate the thyroid, pituitary, or adrenal glands. Knowing your body's heavy metal loads can be the beginning of a road to better health if you are suffering with symptoms from IBS to thyroid issues to autoimmune conditions and heart disease. This subject is probably best addressed with an integrative medical doctor, but I just wanted to touch on it as an honorable mention about how you can begin or fully address your healing journey.

As a restorative dentist, I can confess that my industry has used amalgam filling material for many decades. Amalgam means a mixture of metals. Amalgam (silvery looking) fillings actually contain fifty percent mercury by molecular weight and then in decreasing order: silver, copper, tin, zinc. The industry as a whole acknowledges that the filling material is toxic waste when removed from a patient's mouth. In some European countries, a dead body cannot be cremated unless these fillings have been removed. Mercury is the concern with these fillings. Mercury loves to bind with sulfur-containing enzymes and hormones in the body. It creates a very heavy bond that is difficult to separate with this chemical and in organ tissue commands your detox pathways and influences your body's reaction to stress. More and more, these amalgams are being phased out of practices as we now have other choices that not only do not have heavy metal burdens but also have the benefit of matching the color of your teeth and allow for more conservative dentistry. It is still an issue if you are having an old amalgam filling removed from your mouth, as mercury is gassed off and inhaled by anyone involved in the removal of a filling – the patient and the members of the dental team.

Please consider seeing a holistic or biological dentist for dental work that involves removing old silver fillings if you want dental work that offers the most protection for your health and can minimize your personal re-exposure and re-absorption into your body of mercury upon amalgam removal.

At my dental office, my team follows the SMART protocol established by the International Association of Oral Medicine and Toxicology (IAOMT) when removing old amalgam fillings to minimize exposure of the patient and the dental team. This protocol also helps to prevent the contamination of our rivers and streams from dental office wastewater run-off.

Cardiovascular Disease, Sleep, and You

Here are some early signs you may see on the face of yourself or of your loved ones that indicate there may be heart troubles brewing:

Xanthelasma: buildup of yellowish fatty deposits around the orbit of the eyes (typically symmetrical presentation around both eyes):

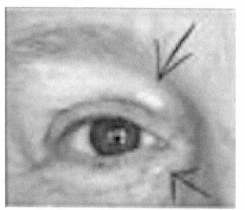 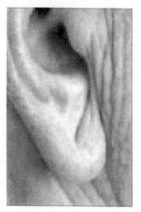

Ear wrinkle: This crease on the ear lobe is another sign of developing cardiovascular issues:

Heart disease includes:

- Hypertension
- Angina
- Arrhythmias
- Heart failure

- Heart attack
- Stroke
- Endocarditis

According to Dr. Mark Houston of Vanderbilt University's Department of Cardiology, the three root causes of vascular disease are imbalance in the body, inflammation, and autoimmune dysfunction. So what he is suggesting is that we now see heart disease as a type of autoimmune disease.[9]

Imbalance occurs when there is an overload of toxins and free radicals, which come from sources external to the body. Again, what one eats and is exposed to environmentally seem to be a potential source for chronic disease. Inflammation will occur in blood vessels as soon as fifteen minutes after a meal is ingested because at this point food that is beginning to be digested will start to be absorbed within the gut into the blood stream. Therefore, inflammation actually begins in the blood vessels just a little after a meal has taken place. Whatever has been ingested will have to be processed by the gut and kidneys to be excreted. Our kidneys are also filters of waste products. When there is toxic overload causing inflammation, the kidneys will begin to have trouble working as a filter over time.

It's too bad we cannot just change our filters in the kidneys like we can change a filter in a car or furnace!

The autoimmune dysfunction piece of vascular biology is going to be turned on when the other processes of the body are not functioning properly. Toxins, which can turn off efficient working of enzymes and hormones and can even bind these same chemicals in the body, can inadvertently cause our body's innate immune fighting ability to turn against us.

Much research in the cardiology world has helped us to understand that if you really wish to predict your cardiovascular system's ability to function efficiently and healthily, one can have your endothelial progenitor cell count computed. The endothelial cell is the cell type lining the interior (the lumen) of all blood vessels. These turn over the lining, regenerating the insides of vessels. The role of the endothelial cell is to generate nitric oxide for the body.[7,8,9,10]

The Nitric Oxide Pathway and Good Sleep

Nitric oxide is a gas that is constantly made by the body. Some stores are in the maxillary sinuses (located behind the cheekbones of the face) and some in the salivary glands surrounding the mouth. Snorers will inadvertently lower their levels of nitric oxide because they are breathing through their mouth, thus changing the ratios of bacteria that live in the mouth. The new bacteria tend to be more problem-causing, contributing to dental disease through cavities and gum disease.

We didn't really know much about nitric oxide's role in the body even just a few years ago. The 1998 Nobel Prize for Medicine was awarded to Furchgott, Ignarro, and Murad for their scientific work determining the Nitric Oxide Pathway. They found that nitric oxide functions as a signaling molecule in the body. It contributes to the turning up or toning down of many biological processes. When you have good levels of this gas being made in the body, your body will function younger and more efficiently. Without strong levels of nitric oxide, it will age more rapidly and tend towards sickness.[10,11]

Inhaling and exhaling through your nose is your best way to increase your body's ability to make nitric oxide. Mouthwashes and a class of digestive medicines for heartburn called H2 blockers (including brand names like Famotidine, Ranitidine, and Cimetidine) can greatly reduce your body's ability to make nitric oxide. In a study by Duke University, chlorhexidine was found to almost completely block the conversion of nitrates to nitrites. In addition, even the weaker (antiseptic and antibacterial) mouthwashes eliminated the effect that nitric oxide had on blood pressure for up to six hours post mouthwash use.[12]

Why Nitric Oxide in the Body Is so Important for Health[11,12]

1. It is the most powerful vasodilator in the body.
2. Its presence prevents plaque, or adhesions, from sticking to the lumen of blood vessels.
3. It enables the remodeling and healing of blood vessels.
4. It creates increased blood flow to the kidneys, encouraging most efficient filtering of salts and water – promotes proper ratios of excretion from the body.
5. It controls the T-cell immune response and reduces inflammation.
6. It encourages formation of lesser amounts of LDL (so called bad cholesterol).
7. It promotes appropriate cell death to weak or abnormal cells (apoptosis).

How Nitric Oxide Is Made and Used in Your Body

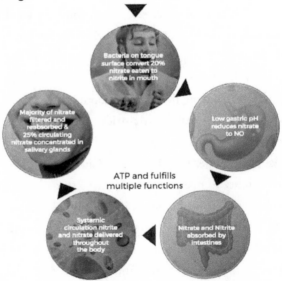

Ultimately low nitric-oxide-making abilities will decrease your body's unit of energy (called ATP), rendering the body literally less energetic. Research also seems to support the concept that a low nitric-oxide-making person may also be more susceptible to a bacterial imbalance (sickness) and therefore will often need to snore more because they have a stuffy nose.

A quick way to try to regain some of the ability to nasal breathe is to try Buteyko breathing exercises. Dr. Konstantin Buteyko was a Ukrainian physiologist practicing in the early part of the twentieth century. He realized that when we breathed through our nose, we tended towards a more regular exchange of air volume, and we had more consistent rations of oxygen to carbon dioxide. He promoted nasal breathing by encouraging people to take a deep inhaled breath in through the nose, hold it for as long as possible, and then for them to slowly exhale it through the nose. After practicing this breathing several times, your nose naturally opens up because your body tries to maintain consistent gas ratios.[13]

If you would like to know how efficient your body is at making nitric oxide to use for the many purposes for which it is needed, consider buying some nitric oxide salivary strips, available on the internet. We routinely will test patients feeling low energy or who have autoimmune disease issues in my dental office with these strips. The test strip will yield a bright pink when exposed to saliva of an efficient nitric oxide maker. But when the body isn't able to convert nitric oxide well, the test strip will remain pale pink or white.

Before the age of forty, the average human can make nitric oxide two different ways:

1. Through the L-Arginine Metabolic pathway using an enzyme called nitric oxide synthase
2. Ingesting green leafy vegetables and beets. This is the only way we make nitric oxide after about the age of forty.

Bacteria in the body and the food you eat enable your ability to make nitric oxide. The bacteria converts the nitrates in foods such as green leafy vegetables and beets or root vegetables into nitrites. This happens in the mouth. The hydrochloric acid levels in the stomach then further reduce nitrites to nitric oxide. Nitrate and nitrite are absorbed in the intestines, and through the blood stream, nitric oxide will be circulated throughout the body. About twenty-five percent of any stored nitric oxide will reside in the salivary glands and some in the maxillary sinus cavities of the skull. We have to make a constant supply of nitric oxide since we cannot store a gas well in the body.[10]

Two types of popular products sold over the counter can drastically reduce your body's ability to make nitric oxide: H2 blockers and anti-bacterial mouthwashes.

So H2 blockers (histamine II blockers of which there were 64.6 million prescriptions written in 2014 in the U.S.A.[10]) block the conversion of nitrites into nitric oxide gas. If your doctor is not following up on your frequency/length of time you use such a classification of drugs, you will suffer from a lack of nitric oxide

And interestingly, mouthwash was a two-trillion-dollar industry in the United States in 2016. Like H2 blockers, we need to consider not using these chronically.

Low levels of nitric oxide are directly linked to hypertension[10] and chronic kidney disease.[11]

If mouthwash and H2 blockers are regularly used, you are basically unnecessarily aging yourself. Digestive troubles and gum inflammation can be managed other ways instead of by these chemicals. I will address these wonderful alternative solutions in the case studies section of this book.

Did you know that bacteria in your mouth circulates throughout your entire body?

In a Finnish study published between 2009 and 2011, autopsies were performed on 101 patients who died from heart attacks. In samples taken of the blood clots causing the heart attacks, it was found that almost seventy-five percent of these contained bacteria associated with tooth decay (streptococcus strains). Also, oral bacteria was circulating in the blood at a rate sixteen times higher than expected. Thirty-five percent of the clots contained bacteria specifically associated with periodontal (gum) disease. The conclusion of this study was that fifty percent of heart attacks were possibly triggered by mouth infections.[30]

In summary, breathing through your nose, maximizing your body's ability to make nitric oxide through a diet of green leafy vegetables, and not using products habitually that block your ability to make nitric oxide will promote more energy and reduce your likelihood of snoring.

Diabetes and Kidney Disease

Any time that you have high blood sugar, as will occur with unchecked diabetes, your body will try to urinate out your extra blood sugar. This often will lead to a need to urinate during the night. There is a strong correlation of diabetes to poor sleep.[14] Also, an estimated 9.4 % of Americans have diabetes, and this number is on the rise.[15] The bacteria in the gut are different between lean and obese and between diabetic and non-diabetic patients.[14]

These bacteria are responsible for changing the metabolic processes in the body. They influence your body's insulin resistance.[16,17] Causes of insulin resistance include genetic predisposition, poor lifestyle, environmental burden, micro-biome imbalances, and altered body composition.[16,18] Again, we see a chicken or the egg relationship between poor sleep and diabetes.

The same tendency repeats with chronic kidney disease and poor sleep. Eighty percent of patients with end stage renal disease suffer daytime sleepiness. They also have an increased stimulation to their sympathetic nervous system while sleeping. Their blood pressure falls while sleeping to abnormally low levels, and this causes an increase in the plasma renin activity and aldosterone (a stress hormone). Research suggests that this situation causes the kidney disease to progress rapidly. These patients do not get much slow-wave sleep (Stages 3 or 4 (REM) sleep). Also, it has been noted that the melatonin that typically regulates the sleep/wake rhythm is not secreted at a regular level in comparison to patients without kidney disease, which results in daytime sleepiness because the patient is not sleeping deeply at night. Fifty to sixty percent of patients who have end stage renal disease have a sleep apnea.[19]

In summary, if you sleep better, your body is healthier. A healthier body will be more able to sustain and postpone development of chronic disease processes that are inflammatory in nature. Maintaining an anti-inflammatory diet is one of the best ways to prevent inflammation. An anti-inflammatory diet is one that contains foods rich in low-glycemic foods such as vegetables and some fruits. The anti-inflammatory diet can also be comprised of lean meats, poultry, eggs, and some whole grains. Other similar variations of the anti-inflammatory diet include the DASH (Dietary Approaches to Stop Hypertension) and Mediterranean diets. Exercise needs to also be an essential component for a lifestyle aimed at warding off disease.

Having vitamins in the abundance that your body needs to function is another step to staying well and sleeping your best. We will explore vitamins and supplements essential for sleep in a later chapter of this book.

Osteoporosis

A study has been completed to determine that poor sleep quality seems to be a lifestyle factor that could influence the severity of osteoporosis in the aging adult.[20]

Parkinson's Disease

Patients with Parkinson's disease are noted for having fragmented REM sleep, a condition called rapid eye movement sleep behavior disorder (RBD). Parkinson's patients have a dysregulation of the dopamine-serotonin network. Also, most patients with Parkinson's disease suffer from excessive daytime sleepiness (EDS). It seems that the go-to pharmaceutical drug for treating the muscle contraction of Parkinson's also may contribute to the difficult sleep these patients have. The poor sleep has been linked to high rates of depression in Parkinson's patients. Diagnosing other sleep issues and having a bedtime routine may help prevent a worsening of sleep.[21]

Depression

Depression is certainly made worse by sleep disorders, and sleep disorders may lead to depression in some individuals. Ninety percent of patients who claim depression also report sleep issues. Two thirds experience insomnia, and forty percent experience difficulty falling asleep and staying asleep or waking too early in the morning. Fifteen percent of patients suffering from depression require more than average amounts of sleep. Chronic insomnia can pre-date the onset of depression, even beginning years before depression takes effect. Also, over half of patients who are statistically diagnosed with depression report insomnia, with eighteen percent of those diagnosed having sleep-disordered breathing. So if you are depressed, please get sleep tested![22]

Cancer

Generally, the way that sleep in relation to cancer has been studied has been a focus on a variety of symptoms regarding poor sleep in patients who have cancer. What is not known are statistics on who develops caner and correlations to underlying sleep conditions. What is known is that poor sleep is a known problem in those that have cancer.[28] What is also known is that often patients who develop cancer have sleep apnea.[29]

Recapping the Main Idea

Reducing gut inflammation will ultimately lead to better sleep and therefore better health. When the gut is left unchecked and in a state of imbalance, inflammation occurs, and we tend to develop chronic disease; the chances of a good night's sleep decrease. Types of diseases associated with this road to bad sleep include obesity, cardiovascular disease, diabetes, kidney disease, osteoporosis, Parkinson's disease, depression, and autoimmune issues. Since the mouth is a window into overall health, inflammation and knowing early signs and symptoms of chronic disease in the mouth could really help you become aware of disease in your body to catch your troubles before they wreck your health.

Sleep issues correspond with chronic inflammation issues, and being aware and preventative could be very helpful towards you staying well.

How can you reduce inflammation in your body? By trying to eat more whole grains and non-processed foods. We could read many other books on this subject, but in a nutshell, below is a list of supplements that can curb your inflammation. Many of these can also reset cholesterol numbers and give you a feeling of more energy. Please check these with your physician to ensure that your personal health is being monitored whenever you consider taking supplements regularly.

***

Supplements

I can attest that many of my dental patients have found great success with supplements.[6]

Fish Oil with a greater ratio of EPA to DHA fatty acids is preferred. You will be less likely to have rancid oil if you can tolerate the liquid oil. For vegans, a eukaryotic version of EPA to DHA fatty acids can be substituted. A dose of 2000 mg daily is suggested. After stopping fish oil for about six weeks, the anti-inflammatory benefits will have dwindled.

Resveratrol is a component of red wine. Limit yourself to one glass nightly or choose a 250 mg daily supplement for this chemical which can reduce LDLs and mildly lower blood pressure. Resveratrol can improve endothelial function (the blood vessels will be healthier, less atherosclerotic).

Berberine functions like a mild metformin and therefore has blood sugar lowering effects. It's helpful to take 250 mg/day. Eat food with berberine. Do not take if you take pharmaceuticals with very specific dosages, as berberine affects the cytochrome p450 pathway of processing pharmaceuticals in the liver. This means the benefit of your pharmaceutical can be altered.

Green Tea contains the active chemical EGCG (epigallocatechin-3-gallate). This is a compound called a catechin. For those who have the COMT gene SNP, EGCG can make those individuals feel irritable. Gene SNP patterns are explained better in the next chapter. Typical dosing if taken in capsule form is 500 mg twice daily. Green tea has blood pressure lowering effects, can lower your LDL levels, and can reduce effects of the Apo B gene.

Niacin: This is the only vitamin B that has a published daily limit. If you take a dose over the limit, you can cause health issues. Start with 100 mg/day. Check with your physician on amounts. Flushing, or a temporary reddening of tissues, can happen while your body adjusts to niacin. Niacin can lower LDL, reduce the LDL particle number, increase HDL, and lower Apo B.

Niacin dosing (through a diet that is low in red and processed meat) has also been linked to a reduction in skin cancer in pilots in a medical study.[23]

Vitamin E can lower effects of Apo B, lower LDL, and raise HDL numbers. Take 100 mg in the evening.

Magnesium relaxes smooth muscle and improves vitamin D and calcium absorption. Take 400 mg citrate or glycinate forms before bed.

Vitamin C: 500 mg twice daily can have blood pressure lowering and wound healing effects. Vitamin C is also great for preventing bleeding gums. Scurvy was suffered by sailors back the days of crews sailing the oceans for years on end where a diet filled with vitamin C containing foods (citrus fruits for example) could not always be provided.

Vitamin D: More on this in the next chapter. It can have blood pressure lowering effects. This vitamin may have the biggest impact on your sleep quality.

Probiotics can alter gut flora and indirectly influence inflammation. Do not take at the same time as berberine as it can cause stomach upset in combination.

Herbs for Inflammation

Ginger, turmeric and boswelli (aka frankincense) can have wonderful anti-inflammatory effects. All of these are found in capsule form. Ginger and turmeric can be grated and sprinkled over foods for savory cooking. If using capsules of turmeric or vast quantities of the fresh root, be aware that turmeric in high doses can affect absorption of pharmaceutical drugs, so again, please let your healthcare provider know if you choose to regularly dose with turmeric.

Protect Your Gut, and You Will Have Your Best Chance to Sleep Better:

With leaky gut, you become unable to efficiently absorb vitamins. Particularly, the levels of vitamins absorbed in the intestines will be affected, which will be covered in the next chapter.

Start the Change of Good Health for Yourself: Know the Basic Good Numbers of Health

When the numbers below are in more optimal ranges, you will also sleep better, generally speaking, because all health issues are chicken or the egg in relation to sleep.

Good Health
Know Your Good Health Numbers.

Total Cholesterol	< 200 mg/dL
HDL-2B (most protective form)	Above 40 mg/dL, men; above 50 mg/dL women
HDL-3 (protective vs. CHD)	
Lipoprotein	Less than 30 mg/dL
Apolipoprotein B (deposits chol. in artery walls)	Less than 60 mg/dL
LDL particle number (better than LDL-C)	Less than 900 particles per mg/dL
VLDL or Triglycerides	Below 75 mg/dL
Vitamin D	At least 30 ng/dL (70+ better)
BMI	< 25
Waist line men < 40"	Waist line women < 35"
Fasting blood glucose HbA1c < 5.7%	Fasting blood sugar < 100 mg/dL

Blood pressure less than 120/90, 110/80 ideal standard.

Aging Occurs Without Exercise and Sleep

It has been noted by many peoples through centuries that better sleep is gained by exercise. Sleep functions as a way for the body to conserve energy so that it may have energy to use when needed during waking hours, when the body may need immediate physical pick-up energy or mental energy to solve a task. Exercise is the best way to work off calories, to release the good feel of endorphins, and is a great way to fight insomnia.[24] Exercise is also a way to fight down inflammation.[25] Aging can also be slowed by exercise.[26] Aging is related to sleep.[27] Exercise and sleep are related to how well we age.

When we exercise, we sleep better. With both of these essential lifestyle processes well practiced, we age better.[27]

Prevention for Aging and a Poor Night's Rest

The old adage is that an ounce of prevention is worth a pound of cure. Eating an anti-inflammatory diet, keeping our weight off with exercise, and simply being aware of how inflammation affects our overall health will take you a long way down the road to a wellness lifestyle.

Exercise can encompass so many varied activities. For some, it can mean getting to the mailbox, while for others it is running a marathon. If you do not currently exercise, then give it a go today!

Smart phone apps, online chat groups, local meetups, and gym memberships can open support doors that suit you.

You will win when you exercise because it will reset how you process your calories. It will help you feel better. You will begin to rest better.

Case Study: Iris with IBS (Irritable Bowel Syndrome)

IBS plagues about twenty percent of the American population every day. As we have explored, there are some chemical, drug, and medical history components such as antibiotic usage that can contribute to the onset of IBS. Also, ingesting foods that have been genetically engineered to sustain weed killers have been linked to IBS, and stress too plays a role in the development of IBS. Since the bacterial flora of the gut is connected and often a disruptive culprit and contributor to the development of IBS, addressing gut health is the answer here. The IBS can contribute to headaches.

Case: Iris, age twenty-seven-years old, was a yoga instructor, previously a literary grad student who was on limited budget. She came in for a dental checkup and reported having IBS and that she had been feeling very stressed. Her IBS episodes would vary between degrees of constipation and diarrhea. She was having frequent and worsening headaches, and her snoring was bothering her husband.

Suggestions:

1. I recommended that Iris keep a food diary to share with her medical practitioner.
2. I told Iris to try an enteric-coated peppermint oil supplement before heavy meals. The enteric coating type should be strongly

suggested over self-made capsules of peppermint oil so that the peppermint oil makes it through the stomach before the capsule breaks down. Peppermint is a natural way to ease digestion.

3. Also, I suggested Iris try tea: peppermint or chamomile teas can ease digestion.

4. If she struggles a lot with stress, Iris may like Bach's Flower Remedy, Agrimony formula. It eases the diarrhea symptoms and helps her process stress that comes from suppressing her feelings (like when one has a history of hiding your true feelings).

5. Magnesium 400 mg (in glycinate form) before bedtime. Magnesium is a muscle relaxer and alleviates constipation. The glycinate form is most easily tolerated. If diarrhea is frequent, then try the ReMag liquid form initially. Magnesium is often a component of pharmaceuticals that treat constipation. Magnesium helps with calcium being absorbed into the bone and also helps create a more relaxed sleep. Better sleep helps a patient manage their life stressors better. Taking magnesium before bed helps the patient to have a bowel movement in the morning, establishing a regularity for this natural daily occurrence.

6. Oregon Grape Root Capsules. I recommend these because this herb helps to close up the tight junctions in the small intestines that have become compromised in the leaky gut. Some patients also take this herb as a gentle, natural preventive medicinal when they are concerned that they are developing a bacterial, viral, or fungal infection as this herb has mild qualities to fight all these invaders of the body. Some research has also shown that Oregon Grape Root capsules can be taken as a mild natural metformin, or in other words, this will lower the blood sugar/insulin response in a pre-diabetic. Since the herb is also antibacterial, it still needs to be determined what the effect to the gut is in the scenario that a patient takes Oregon Grape Root for an

extended period of time. For this reason, I recommended only trying for a few weeks. People on medications that are highly dose-specific should not take Oregon Grape Root capsules or berberine-containing herbs (Goldenseal is another example of this) because the active ingredient in the mechanism of action can inhibit some dose-specific drugs from being absorbed properly by interacting with the CYP pathway in liver metabolism of the drug. I recommended Iris try 250 mg tablets with meals once/day.

7. Turmeric capsules. One capsule of Turmeric is about the equivalent of thirteen fresh teaspoons of turmeric root, available at many grocery stores. There is a craze about turmeric coming from the explosive medical research that has been completed on this herb. I recommended Iris try taking turmeric for IBS symptoms because of its strong anti-inflammatory effect on the body.

8. Probiotics with digestive enzymes and digestive enzymes would be great for Iris. I recommend and have seen many patients improve their IBS frequency when they take enzymes that assist with food digestion and are replenishing/rebuilding the variety of bacterial flora with probiotics. Even taking probiotics a few times weekly can significantly improve the bacteria flora. Do not take probiotics with Oregon Grape Root as this combination together can cause stomach discomfort. The digestive enzymes can also help ease digestion, as many of us do not produce enough stomach acid to digest our food. Dr. Jonathan Aviv's book called *The Acid Watcher's Diet* is a great resource of more information on this topic.

9. To address Iris's snoring, I made her a snore guard. We verified with a take-home sleep test that she did not have sleep apnea but was merely snoring while sleeping on her back.

10. I told Iris to follow up with your primary care doctor of choice. I told her to bring this list of my recommendations to the appointment so the doctor knows what she may have tried at home.

11. Six months later, Iris brought me a pretty pink coffee mug imprinted with the words "You're Gorgeous!" Her headaches and IBS had resolved! Her physician confirmed from the food diary that her IBS was indeed food-related, and she had cut dairy products from her diet. Her gums were healthy again. Her oral appliance was preventing her from snoring, so her sleeping no longer is waking her husband. Success!

In the next chapter, I discuss links between vitamin and mineral levels and how these can affect sleep duration, type of sleep, and sleep quantity. I also delve into the relationships between vitamin and mineral levels and the pharmaceuticals that can deplete one's levels of these nutrients, thus indirectly affecting sleep.

Chapter 6:

Sleep Is Affected by Your Vitamin and Mineral Levels

"One cannot think well, love well, sleep well,
if one has not dined well."
– Virginia Woolf

Poor digestion caused by inflammation, leaky gut, and metabolic syndrome (X or Z forms) can affect sleep because these conditions impact the amount of vitamins and minerals absorbed by the gut. The diagram below shows where in the gut various nutrients are absorbed. When one's digestive system is not functioning optimally, as is the case in at least twenty percent of Americans, the body will have some nutritional deficiency as a result, despite an optimal diet. As a result of our dietary choices and modern diet, Americans often have chronic deficiencies in a number of essential vitamins and nutrients, as seen below:

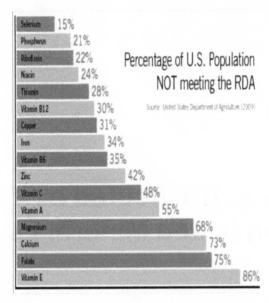

And here is a diagram that shows where in our gut various vitamins and nutrients are absorbed:[2]

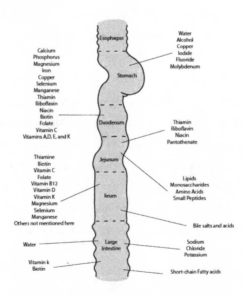

Gene mutations and pharmaceuticals can also be a source of hidden vitamin depletion. How can you know if you are one of these patients? Actually, most people are. Patients who take some of the mainstream pharmaceuticals can experience depletion of vitamins or essential nutrients that can contribute to developing sleep apnea.

People may find they are accidentally potentially running low due to either genetic reasons or pharmaceuticals may decide to supplement.

As Americans, millions of us regularly take a regimen of drugs to treat many varieties of illness, both chronic and temporary, to alleviate symptoms or to treat the condition.

The main vitamins and minerals associated with sleep effects are listed below. Foods that contain these are listed as well. In each description will be the pharmaceuticals that can affect absorption of these nutrients. After reviewing these, we will check out common gene mutations that can also contribute to what vitamins and nutrients you may decide you should supplement through diet or products so you can sleep better.

Vitamin B12

Vitamin B12 treatments have been noted to help people who have irregularly sleep/wake cycles and those suffering from leg cramps.[9,10] A medical study reported that young women who have low vitamin B12 levels are more likely to require longer sleep time.[10,11] Sleep Duration is negatively associated with B12. In other words, taking a B12 supplement will contribute to you not sleeping as long as without the supplement if you have low B12 levels.

Signs of a vitamin B12 deficiency include:[20]

- Weakness, tiredness, dizziness
- Pale skin and gums
- Smooth tongue
- Heart palpitations .
- Vision loss

- Numbness, tingling, muscle weakness, problems walking
- Depression
- Constipation or diarrhea
- More likely to occur with a vegan diet: hyperthyroidism, with other dietary troubles such as Crohn's disease.
- Atrophic gastritis, in which your stomach lining has thinned
- Pernicious anemia, which makes it hard for your body to absorb vitamin B12
- Conditions that affect your small intestine, such as Crohn's disease, celiac disease, bacterial growth, or a parasite
- Immune system disorders, such as lupus or Graves' disease

Foods that contain B12 include:

- Meat, fish, poultry
- Eggs
- Milk
- Fortified breakfast cereal

If you have pernicious anemia or have trouble absorbing vitamin B12, you'll need shots of this vitamin at first. You may need to keep getting these shots, take high doses of a supplement, or get it nasally after that.

Pharmaceuticals That Lower B12 Levels:[25]

- Metformin (for diabetes treatment): take a sublingual or injectable B12 supplement to counter this effect.
- Corticosteroids such as prednisone and Decadron deplete B12 supplies.

Vitamin B6 (Pyridoxine)

Vitamin B6 has been studied in patients who have had a significant emotional loss and are experiencing grief. Because B6 is a cofactor for an enzyme in the biosynthesis pathway for serotonin, a deficiency of B6 is associated with one's ability to make serotonin and receive good sleep.[12,13]

B6 is also helpful to reduce general inflammation. It is involved in over 150 enzyme reactions that help you digest the fat, carbohydrates, and protein ingested. It helps your body to make hemoglobin so that you can absorb iron.[19]

Signs of a vitamin B6 deficiency include:

- Cracked or sore lips
- Skin rashes
- Sore, glossy red tongue
- Moodiness
- Tiredness, low energy (tending towards anemia)
- Tingling and hands and feet
- Seizures
- Weakened immune system
- High homocysteine levels (from protein digestion)

Increased homocysteine levels have been linked with several health issues, most notably heart disease and stroke, as well as Alzheimer's disease. When homocysteine is elevated, it can damage blood vessels and nerves.

Foods That Contain B6:

- Meats: pork, poultry, fish
- Whole grains, oatmeal, brown rice, wheat-germ
- Eggs
- Vegetables
- Soya beans
- Ricotta cheese

You can easily meet your B6 needs with diet.

Pharmaceuticals That Affect B6 Levels:[26]

- Antibiotics of most any kind will deplete this water-soluble vitamin.

- Isoniazid and Seromycin, both used for treating tuberculosis infections, are also attributed to B6 depletion.
- Valproic Acid (Depakote) used to treat depression.
- Levodopa also depletes B6 levels.
- Theophylline for respiratory health is a depletory.
- Clonidine (Catapress) and methyldopa contribute to a B6 deficiency.
- Estrogen replacement therapy can cause lowered B6 levels.

Vitamin D

We get vitamin D primarily through exposure to sunshine. Traditionally in winter months when it is cold (our skin is covered or time is spent indoors) and daylight hours are more limited, we do not typically get as much vitamin D as on summer days spent outdoors. Low amounts of vitamin D are associated with depression and with a weakened immune system. Low serum vitamin D levels are also related to sleep disorders as well as many other poor health conditions including onset of autoimmune disease.

Vitamin D also functions to affect the balance between calcium and phosphate, it affects muscle function, affects the immune response capability, and assists with nerve and heart function.[3,4,5]

Vitamin D deficiency symptoms can appear as or be in co-morbidity with:[5,6]

- Muscle weakness
- Diseases of inflammation covered in the previous chapter, including diabetes and cardiovascular disease, cancer, multiple sclerosis

Poor gut health is related to your body's ability to absorb vitamin D. Healthy fats in the diet help you absorb vitamin D from foods. Healthy fats include natural vegetable oils such as olive oil, flax oil, walnut oil, and coconut oil, and raw butter or ghee. Healthy gut flora promotes better absorption of nutrients in the intestines. Magnesium supplements also help with vitamin D absorption because it is used to make enzymes responsible for absorbing vitamin D from dietary sources. Most Americans are reportedly low in magnesium. If you are low in magnesium, you will not be able to absorb dietary vitamin D. This is why supplementing with magnesium is important if you are low in vitamin D. Dietary vitamin D is absorbed in the jejunum and ileum of the small intestines.

Many vitamin D receptors are located in the brain stem and these are connected to nerve tissue that impacts the stages of sleep. These tissues keep us from moving our bodies during REM sleep.[5] When we are low in vitamin D, our sleep quality cannot be good as our bodies cannot get REM sleep. Low vitamin D levels are also associated with high blood pressure, and supplementing with vitamin D can help lower your blood pressure.[21,22]

Getting your gut in its best shape and possibly supplementing your vitamin D may help resolve some of your sleep issues. We absorb vitamin D naturally through our skin, which delivers it to our liver and kidneys to be converted into the form the body uses called calcitriol. Liquid supplements seem to be best absorbed rather than tablets if you are using a supplement.

These are natural ways to absorb more vitamin D:[5,6]

- Get at least 15 minutes daily of sun
- Darker-skinned individuals need more vitamin D. Because of more melanin, our skin is darker, which blocks more UV-B rays, therefore blocking the absorption of vitamin D
- Consider not wearing sunscreen under make-up if you are limited in your sun exposure.
- You have a harder time absorbing as you age. Make getting time outside more of a priority as you get older.
- Keep in mind that air pollution can block UV-B rays, from which your body makes its vitamin D.

- Know that the farther you live from the equator impacts how many UV-B rays available for you.
- Not many foods contain vitamin D, and it is hard to eat enough through diet alone. Fish (about seven ounces) and mushrooms (about six ounces of portabella mushroom) are natural food sources of vitamin D. Milk products are often fortified with vitamin D.

Vitamin D Food Source	IUs per serving
High Vitamin Cod Liver Oil, 1tsp	1,150
Standard Cod Liver Oil, 1tsp	400
Salmon, cooked, 3.5 oz	360
Mackerel, cooked, 3.5 oz	345
Tuna, canned in oil, 3 oz	200
Sardines, canned in oil, drained, 1.75 oz	250
Egg Yolk	20
Beef Liver, cooked, 3.5 oz	15
Cheese, Swiss, 1 oz	12

Source: National Institute of Health 2009

Even with sunlight, it can be difficult to receive all the vitamin D you need. Supplementing from food sources is helpful to ensure you have enough.

A vitamin D serum level of less than 20 ng/mL on tests were most highly associated with sleep disorders in a meta-analysis of the relationship of vitamin D and sleep disorders. Generally, vitamin D levels are considered low at a threshold of 30 ng/mL, although levels over 70 ng/mL are much more optimal.

Supplements for vitamin D come in two forms: D2 and D3. D2 is also called ergocalciferol and comes from yeasts and mushrooms. D3 is called cholecalciferol and is sourced from fish and animals. D3 seems to be absorbed more easily and has been found to help stabilize a deficiency more quickly than D2 supplementation.

In dentistry, we can determine a so-called "chair sign" in a patient with a vitamin D deficiency on an x-ray.

Below is an x-ray showing "normal pulp chambers" which would suggest a normal vitamin D level.[21]

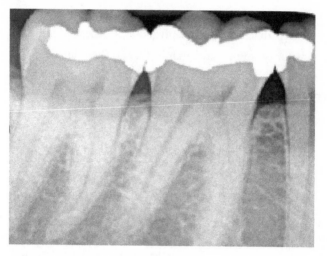

Below is an x-ray showing "chair shaped pulp/nerve chambers" in the lower back molars which would suggest a low vitamin D level.[21]

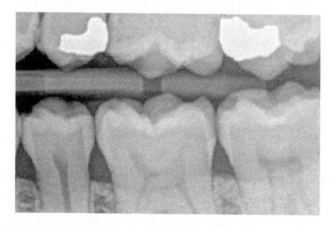

A dentist should be involved with a team effort for detecting daytime and sleep-time habits where teeth and bite are analyzed.

There are pharmaceutical drugs that interfere with vitamin D:[23]

- Lipid-lowering effects of statin drugs are disabled with Vitamin D.
- The antibacterial effect of medicines for tuberculosis are also affected by D.
- Laxatives affect Vitamin D absorption levels through the intestines in a negative way.
- Drugs that activate the pregnane X receptor can lead to deficiency symptoms in Vitamin D, and these include:

Drugs That Activate the Pregnane-X-receptor (PXR)[23]

PXR-Ligands	Examples
Antiepileptic drugs	Phenytoin, Carbamazepine
Antineoplastic drugs	Cyclophophamide, Taxol, Tamoxifen
Antibiotics	Clotrimazole, Rifampicin
Anti-inflammatory agents	Nifedipine, Spironolactone
Antiretroviral drugs	Ritononavir, Saquinavir
Antihypertensives	Nifedipine, Spironolactone
Endocrine drugs	Cyproterone acetate
Herbal medicines	Kava kava, St. Johns wort

Multiple Sclerosis: Patients with M.S. often have been given glucocorticoid therapy regimens for M.S. treatment, and these patients often have osteoporosis as a direct result of the interaction with Vitamin D.

Breast Cancer: Patients low in Vitamin D may have worse muscle and skeletal pain associated with therapy due to aromatase inhibitor interactions with Vitamin D when estrogen levels fall. Also, prognosis for women suffering from breast cancer was worsened if their level of serum D levels was less than 20 ng/mL. These cancer patients also have more likelihood of oral ulcers because of the vitamin D deficiency. These patients also have been shown to have bone damage post cancer treatment that is worsened with low vitamin D levels.

Iron: Low iron levels have been found to shorten sleep duration in adults and infants. With iron deficiency anemia, infants are more likely to wake up during the night, sleep less time, and have delayed onset of non-REM sleep spindles which affects REM sleep too. This trend may even set the infant up for altered patterns between Stage 4 (REM) and Stage 3 sleep. Iron deficiency anemia in adults is attributed to less sleep and altered sleep stages.

Signs of Low Iron:[17]

- Extreme fatigue
- Weakness
- Pale skin
- Chest pain, fast heartbeat, or shortness of breath
- Headache, dizziness
- Cold hands and feet
- Bald/red tongue
- Brittle nails

Foods Containing Iron:[18]

- Spinach and other green leafy vegetables (non-heme iron-not from blood source)
- 3 oz. of meat
- Fortified breakfast cereal
- ½ cup tofu
- 1/2 cup beans
- 1/4 cup wheat germ
- 1 oz. pumpkin or squash seeds

* 1/2 cup raisins

Pharmaceuticals That Lower Iron Levels:[26]
* Levothyroxine (Levothyroid, Levoxyl) will lower iron levels
* Cimetidine (Tagamet), famotidine (Pepcid), ranitidine (Zantac)

Magnesium

Magnesium is one of my personal favorite recommended supplements for helping with sleep. I call magnesium the six-dollar sleep solution.

Magnesium has an effect on sleep duration and increases quiet sleep and decreases active sleep. In infants, a conversation needs to be held with a pediatrician because dosages can affect sleep patterns that potentially influence infant sleep patterns for years. Expectant mothers taking magnesium sulfate had more active sleep without REM. In the elderly, magnesium supplements apparently have been found to reverse age-related sleep changes (less REM), but more studies are needed to fully appreciate the effects of magnesium in the elderly.[13]

Magnesium also alleviates constipation and helps absorption of calcium into bone tissue.

Indications of Low Magnesium Levels:
* Muscle Soreness, spasms or tightness, convulsions
* Headaches, weakness, dizziness
* PMS
* Mood problems, hallucinations
* Fatigue
* Irregular heartbeats and insomnia

Foods Containing Magnesium:
* Dark chocolate (yay!)
* Avocado

- Nuts
- Legumes
- Tofu
- Pumpkin, Flax, Chia seeds
- Whole grains
- Salmon, mackerel, halibut
- Bananas
- Leafy green vegetables

Other Ways to Ingest Magnesium:

- Epsom salts baths (magnesium sulfate)
- Tablets: glycinate (easiest on the stomach), sulfate or citrate

Pharmaceuticals That Affect Magnesium Levels:[24,25,26]

1. Proton Pump Inhibitors such as omeprazole, lansonprazole, ritonavir: These are widely used for gastric-acid related disorders and cause depleted magnesium levels because they reduce stomach acid, and magnesium is digested because of stomach acid in the stomach. P.P.I.s reduce stomach production by as much as 95%. These drugs also affect calcium absorption by way of affecting magnesium absorption.[25] Please do not take PPI's for long time periods.

2. Patients taking loop and thiazide diuretics will more easily pee out their magnesium.

3. Potassium retaining agents: amiloride, triamterene and spironolactone

4. In patients using digoxin, magnesium helps prevent cardiac arrhythmias. Magnesium helps prevent atrial fibrillation in digoxin users. But in patients who have congestive heart failure, digoxin can prevent absorption of magnesium with reabsorption of magnesium in patients leading to a life-threatening problem.

5. Corticosteroids can deplete magnesium levels.

6. Estrogen therapy can contribute to lessened magnesium levels.

Zinc and Copper

Zinc and Copper have an inverse absorption relationship. Low levels of zinc shorten sleep duration.

Generally speaking, zinc supplementation is helpful for building immune system protection from common colds. Zinc is also helpful for fighting depression, anorexia. Symptoms of low zinc include:[13,14,15,16]

- Inability to smell or taste
- Hypothyroidism
- Fatigue
- Brittle nails, hair loss, dry skin, and hair
- Lowered sex drive in women and Erectile Dysfuntion (E.D.) in men

Foods Containing Copper and Zinc:[13,14,15,16]

- Meat
- Shellfish
- Legumes (peas and beans)
- Seeds
- Nuts
- Diary
- Eggs
- Whole Grains

Indications of low zinc levels include a poor sense of smell. A home test for zinc can be conducted using a bottle of liquid zinc sulfate using a concentration of 1 gm/L of water. Next, taste the solution. Depending on the severity of the taste, you will have an idea of your level. Your doctor can confirm the level if you want to be exact.

1. If you are very deficient, the solution will taste like water. If you test this way, most try supplementing with over 150 mg/day for several months and then retest later.

2. If you have a metallic aftertaste, you are fairly deficient in zinc. Try supplementing but with a lesser amount, perhaps 100 mg/day. Retest after several months.

3. A slight deficiency is suggested if you begin to experience a metallic taste about ten seconds after swallowing. Consider supplementing with 50 mg/day.

4. When the body is not zinc deficient, the solution will taste very unpleasant. A dosage of 15-25 mg/day is typically good for this person but can be dosed up to 100 mg/day if the person is experiencing stress or if they are exposed to an infection.

5. If there is too much zinc when tested, your stomach will be slightly upset after you tested positive for no deficiency.

Indications of Low Copper Levels:

- Fatigue
- Problems with memory or learning
- Sensitivity to cold
- Pale Skin
- Premature gray hair
- Weak/brittle bones
- Frequent illness
- Difficulty walking
- Vision loss
- Slow wound healing
- Loss of taste
- Sexual dysfunction

Pharmaceuticals That Affect Copper and Zinc Levels:[13,14,15,16,26]

- Ethambutol (Myambutol) used to treat tuberculosis.
- Corticosteriods (prednisone) can deplete zinc supplies.
- Zinc depletion is connected to ACE inhibitor drugs, including benazepril (Lotensin), captopril (Capoten), enalapril (Vasotec), fosinopril (Monopril), lisinopril (Prinivil, Zestril), quinapril (Accupril), ramipril (Altace).
- Chlorthiazide (Diuril), hydrochlorothiazide (Microzide) are linked to zinc deficiency.
- Cimetidine (Tagamet), famotidine (Pepcid), and ranitidine (Zantac) lower zinc levels.

***

Sleep duration is negatively associated with B12, Cu, and K. Sleep duration is positively associated with levels of Fe, Zn, and Mg. To know that your levels of these nutrients are within a normal range and/or to account for losses due to diet choices or pharmaceuticals can be an inexpensive way to regulate one's sleep.

Also, please shop for organic leafy green vegetables whenever possible. Non-organic greens are potentially very high in pesticide residue.

Gene SNP's: A New Medical Cause-Effect Treatment Paradigm

Gene "SNP" is an abbreviation for Single Nucleotide Polymorphism. In the last twenty years, scientists have begun to decode the human genome, breaking down an individual's gene to determine its direct influence on how the body works. Most of the population has a number of these mutations in their DNA that are significant to change how you live but are not life threatening in themselves as a chromosome problem could potentially be. At least hundreds of gene SNPs have been studied, and we will only be able to cover some of the main ones in this book.

Lifestyle choices seem to turn the effect of gene SNPs or increase their influence on us in terms of health. The importance of Gene SNPs in this book about sleep solutions is that you need to know if you have some of the essential ones because the existence of these in your DNA can cause you to not absorb vitamins well and to reduce your body's capability to handle inflammation or stress or to detox. Remember that when you have higher inflammation loads or reduced vitamin and mineral supplies, your sleep will be affected. We are also discovering that there are at least a couple of gene SNPs that directly influence sleep.

Medical research is exploding in the field of Gene SNP's, and some of the research findings are controversial. In summary, I believe it is wise for every patient to have been tested. You have the test completed once, and this will gain you a lifetime of information. If you are not positive once, you will never need to consider this as an influencer of how you can heal.

SNPs can also affect how we absorb our nutrients. There are several gene SNPs that are related to inflammation or are directly related to sleep.

Below is a diagram that links many of these various metabolic SNP pathways together. The pathways are depicted in the boxes, and they function rather like cogs in an old-fashioned clock. When one pathway wheel does not function efficiently, the wheel grinds slowly. Ultimately, these wheels feed the NOS (nitric oxide pathway) and the Krebs Cycle (that is responsible for your body making energy, or ATP).

Here is a visual that shows how a number of common gene SNPs are related to symptoms of poor health. Many of these genes spin pathways, rather like cogs in a clock mechanism. When one of the cogs is slow, then the wheel does not spin optimally. In the diagram below, enzymatic pathways are listed, including vitamins and supplements (shown in ovals) necessary for the cog to turn. When you have a gene SNP (or a number of these), being aware of which vitamins or supplements you can potentially take can ease the slow cog and thus move your body's metabolism along in a more optimal way. Best health can be achieved with these processes working optimally. Best sleep will also be easier to obtain when these wheels spin optimally.

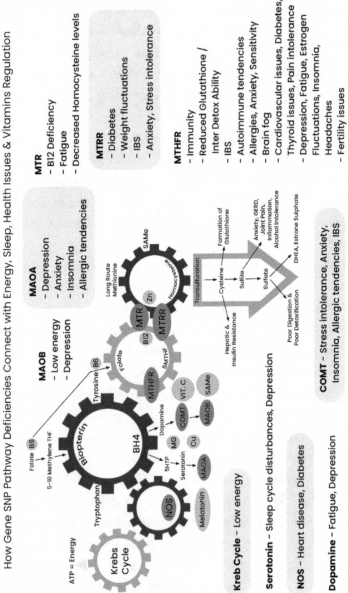

How Gene SNP Pathway Deficiencies Connect with Energy, Sleep, Health Issues & Vitamins Regulation

The figure depicts many commonly researched gene SNPs and the health symtoms of when they are not functionally optimally.

Some common SNPs related to the body not being able to detox easily in liver or kidney pathways cause alterations in the homocysteine levels of the body. The state of having an imbalance of homocysteine creates increased whole-body inflammation. This happens because the body cannot absorb some of the nutrients needed to add to the efficiency of these detoxification pathways. Two gene SNPs that are major contributors to the inflammation load in the body are:

MTHFR: Sometimes referred to as Mother-Father Gene and stands for Methylenetetrahydrofolate reductase. This enzyme converts homocysteine into methionine. When this pathway is not working efficiently because the gene is present or amplified through lifestyle choices and stress, the result is that there are higher levels of homocysteine. This is the most studied of the SNPs. There are two major groupings under the MTHFR gene umbrella: 1298AC and 677CT. Approximately over fifty percent of the population in the USA is positive for MTHFR. Native Americans are ninety percent positive for MTHFR gene. MTHFR is both a reference to a metabolic pathway and is an enzyme in this pathway. It is responsible for how we absorb many of the B vitamins including: B2 (riboflavin), B9 (folic acid), and B12. To help your body counter the effects of the MTHFR gene, supplementation with vitamins is often very helpful. Supplementing with vitamins that are pre-loaded with what the body lacks facilitate the MTHFR pathway.

Specifically, MTHFR people benefit from a supplement cocktail including:

- Methylated folate (Vitamin B9)
- Methylcobalamine (B12 with a cobalt atom added)
- Riboflavin (Vitamin B2)
- Vitamin C
- Zinc

How much and more specifics on how you should consider supplementing should be reviewed with your physician, although your dentist should also be able to have a conversation with you. Patients with MTHFR are much more likely to have periodontal disease because of the body's increased inflammatory load that will be always somewhat present when you are a MTHFR gene carrier.

MAOA, MAOB, MTR, and MTRR are closely related due to the close relationship with MTHFR enzyme pathway, so these are demonstrated separately in the diagram but are not elaborated upon in separate sections here.

COMT stands for Catechol-O-methyltransferase and is also a pathway and an enzyme. This enzyme breaks down or deactivates catecholamines such as dopamine, epinephrine, and norepinephrine. It is another pathway that contributes to a potential build up in inflammatory chemicals such as homocysteine. It is linked to a woman's ability to dump extra estrogens as she approaches menopause and continues into the next phases of her life. Buildup of these higher estrogens is linked to breast cancer in some women. It is also connected to increased states of anxiety when this gene SNP is amplified by lifestyle choices. In other words, when this pathway is not highly functioning, it is difficult for the individual to bring the body into a physical and emotional state of equilibrium when faced with a stressor. As much as eighty percent of the population may have a gene variant of the COMT pathway. COMT is produced in the brain, liver, kidneys, and blood. When the pathway is not functioning or producing enough of this enzyme, the individual can feel more like worrying instead of warrior-ing. This person ends up carrying stress chemicals in their system longer than they would if COMT pathway functioned ideally. They can more easily become depressed or have substance abuse issues, anger, and impulsivity since their dopamine levels are lower than normal.

Patients who are heterozygous (from one parent) or homozygous (have the SNP from both parents) COMT gene SNP benefit from taking:

- SAMe supplement
- Magnesium
- Vitamin D
- NAC (n-Acetylcholine)

SAMe is the abbreviation for S-adenosyl-L-methionine, and this is a chemical the body makes. SAMe helps produce and regulates hormones and protects cell membranes. It is taken as a supplement for treating depression, liver trouble, and osteoarthritis. It can interact with antidepressant medication, so taking SAMe needs to be discussed with your physician if you already take an anti-depressant and want to try SAMe. Also, do not mix SAMe with antipsychotics, amphetamines, the cold medicine dextromethorphan, narcotics, or St. John's Wort because mixing these with SAMe can cause serotonin syndrome (a buildup of serotonin which can lead to psychotic episodes).

SAMe is typically taken in a dose of 400 mg up to 1600 mg for depression symptoms. Check with your doctor for a dose that best suits you.

A diet that has more flavanoids (found in red wine, berries) and quercetin (found in red onions, peppers, apples, grapes, black tea, and broccoli) help support health in patients who have the COMT gene SNP variations. Quercetin has anti-inflammatory effects. Flavanoids have strong antioxidant activity, which supports eliminating extra estrogens that occur in patients with COMT gene (preventing breast cancer in females). In males, COMT gene has more effect on liver function.[29]

NOS Pathway is an abbreviation for the Nitric Oxide Pathway. The ability to make NOS efficiently is perhaps one of the best ways to stay healthier and younger. Easing the pathway by assisting the other common gene SNPs is helpful to your NOS functioning well in your body because when you take inflammation off the table of health, you have fewer complications to stay healthy. For example, if you have gene SNPs for either or both MTHFR and COMT and you have diminished their influence on your metabolism, your NOS Pathway has a stronger likelihood of not being affected by these gene SNPs associated with inflammation.

To check how well you make nitric oxide, salivary test strips can be purchased on the internet. If you are low, Neo 40 tablets or eating high nitrate foods (such as beets) can be taken to increase the level you make. Also reducing usage of proton pump inhibitors and mouthwash frequency can help.

CLOCK SNP rs2070062 is an abbreviation for Circadian Locomotor Output Cycles Protein Kaput (not pictured), and it regulates turning on a molecular circadian rhythm clock, which influences a number of other metabolic pathways. In particular, it has been studied and linked to an increased BMI because of CLOCK's influence on sleep duration and quality as well as levels of adiponectin and leptin. Those who have and have amplified the CLOCK SNP rs2070062 have shorter duration of sleep whereas those who have CLOCK SNP rs6853192 sleep longer. Those who have CLOCK variant rs207006 sleep for a shorter than average amount of time. It has been found that the BMI in those who are carriers for CLOCK SNPs rs6820823, rs3792603, and rs11726609 is lower than the average population and that those with this gene SNP sleep longer. It has also been determined that there is a genetic link between genes that set circadian rhythm and influencers of obesity, but this link is not fully understood yet.[27]

The diabetes risk variant MTNR1B (not pictured) influences sleep, circadian rhythm, and melatonin physiology. More studies are needed, but what is understood is that when this gene SNP is present, the relationship between mealtime with to melatonin levels and bedtime may influence the development of diabetes Type II (T2D) in the patient. In other words, in a scenario when a MTNR1B gene SNP patient has higher melatonin levels and eats close to bedtime, a change takes place in the body's circadian rhythm which causes decreased glucose tolerance and leads towards Type II diabetes onset.[27]

An anti-inflammatory diet and low glycemic foods (foods low in sugar) will help minimize this gene SNP.[28]

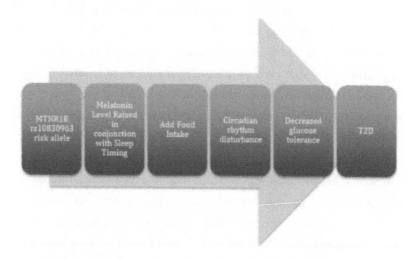

How to Get Yourself Tested for SNP's

SNPs can be identified through a blood test or salivary test. Initially, 23 and Me had SNP results listed in the information sent back to clients. Nowadays, this is back in the hands of professionals. My vote is to go with a salivary test, and medical, chiropractic, naturopathic, or dental providers can provide this screening test. It takes about two weeks for results to come back to the patient, and the cost will vary from $120 to several hundred dollars, depending on the numbers of SNPs tested.

Gene SNP testing is not commonly offered in most parts of the USA, but testing is easy to accomplish. The information potentially gleaned from gene SNP testing can truly help the individual prevent onset of future disease processes. I encourage everyone to consider purchasing this test. The cost will most likely be out-of-pocket. I don't find this surprising because I personally expect to look out for myself rather than have a medical insurance plan look out for my overall health. If you wish to be tested for gene SNPs, ask your provider.

The Patient Who Has Trouble Sleeping – Marie (COMT and MTHFR Gene Carrier)

Marie, age forty-two, was a single mom of a diabetic elderly dog, and she had trouble sleeping. Part of the issue is that her dog had diabetes, so she ensured care for the dog by maintaining a schedule to care for the dog. This meant that even on really late nights or early starts of days, she would arrange her sleep and living schedule around the canine, who really was such a lovely creature! Marie had been so stressed about her job and life path. She had recently left a hard-driving corporate job to pursue dreams of running her own company. She made many lifestyle changes that were filled with new happy habits such as daily yoga and walks and jogs outside, but she was stressed with the uncertainty that came with running her fledgling business. Marie was also seeking a correction for her crowded teeth.

Suggestions for Marie

Marie was salivary tested and found to have both MTHFR and COMT gene SNPs. She also wanted to lose weight. She had been exhausted for months. These were also considered in formulating the following treatment plan:

1. Try the Adrenal failure regimen (which is covered in the case study at the end of the next chapter).
2. To sleep better, consider Passionflower tea to ease the burden of being a caregiver. Passionflower was found to ease the mind, drinking 2-3 cups of tea regularly.
3. Other teas geared more towards sleep: Valerian herbal tea, hops tea for a stronger sleep effect. Try chamomile for children or for a mild sleep aid. If using Valerian, do not mix with barbiturates or other sleep medication or antidepressants as it will enhance the effects of the medication and sleep will be more pronounced.

4. Another herb to try (not necessarily with Valerian) would be skullcap. Skullcap is an herb traditionally used to improve sleep and gives the feeling of someone removing your worries whilst sleep. Skullcap can be taken over the counter as either a tincture or capsule.

5. For the MTHFR, take a methylated B12 and methylated folic acid complex that contains the other vitamin B's as well as a zinc/vitamin C supplement daily. For COMT, reduce intake/avoid green tea as this can contribute to feelings of irritability in a COMT gene SNP patient. Also, a COMT patient may benefit from SAMe as a supplement for mood elevation. A SAMe dose of 400 mg can be started since Marie is not on any other medications. Marie can also increase her dietary intake of foods containing flavonoids (berries for example) and quercetin (green leafy vegetables and red onions) to minimize unwanted effects of COMT gene SNP.

6. Encourage Marie to exercise daily and to continue to connect socially with others in her community.

7. We sent Marie home with a home sleep test and it was found to be negative for sleep disordered breathing. Marie was found to not be actively grinding her teeth. Clear aligners were made to straighten her teeth, and active treatment was completed within six months.

Chapter 7:

Links Between Hormones and Sleep

"That we are not much sicker and much madder than we are is due exclusively to that most blessed and blessing of all natural graces, sleep."
– Aldous Huxley

ormones in the body can also affect sleep. These sleep effects are different for females and males.

Women's Hormones and Sleep

Progesterone and estrogen levels affect sleep. Both hormones actually influence contraction of the genioglossus muscle (a tongue muscle). This prevents airway collapse during sleep. Progesterone also stabilizes breathing during sleep through increasing the urge to breathe. This means that in a surge of progesterone in the luteal phase of the menstrual cycle (between a period but before ovulation) compared to the follicular phase, there is increased risk of upper airway collapse, thus more sleep issues.[1,2]

Especially in the mouth breather where carbon dioxide levels are not normalized (fall less than 6% carbon dioxide), high progesterone levels can predispose a patient to periodic breathing and UARS. Supplementing with testosterone in these women can increase their apneic threshold, meaning that their sleep apnea symptoms worsen.[1]

Pregnancy, Polycystic Ovary Syndrome (PCOS), and Menopause Are Conditions That Can Increase the Frequency of Snoring and Sleep Issues

There are different hormonal states between these three conditions potentially affecting a woman. In pregnancy, estrogen and progesterone levels are generally elevated. In PCOS, there is too much androgen chemical, a precursor for estrogen, that has not formed into female hormone.[1]

Pregnancy: During pregnancy, ten to forty-give percent of women are reported to snore, and this statistic rises in women suffering pre-eclampsia (an extremely stressed state of being just before an imminent birth when both the mother and baby are in a very dangerous situation from toxins) to seventy-five percent. Sleep apnea is statistically much more prevalent in women who are obese. In the first trimester, ten percent of obese women have sleep apnea, and almost a third are apniac by the third trimester. The weight gain, extra fluid, and hormones present during pregnancy seem to drive up the risk of OSA.[1]

The rising risk of OSA in an expectant mom is a huge concern for the developing baby because the OSA is definitely linked to lesser growth of the uterus, and this may play a role in development of gestational diabetes, preterm delivery, hypertension in the mother, and pre-eclampsia. Increased sympathetic nervous system stimulus also develops in the expectant mother with OSA that is untreated.[1]

Side sleeping has been found to help pregnant women to sleep best during pregnancy.

In the case of pre-eclampsia, the woman with OSA often has a low breathing rate, low AHI score, increased carbon dioxide levels, but has developed more episodes of decreased oxygen saturation during REM sleep. These conditions lead to hypertension, fluid retention, increased sympathetic nervous system activation, and ultimately create an environment that predisposes the mother to pre-eclampsia. CPAP has been studied and found to be a helpful treatment for this situation to aid health of the mother and the baby.[1]

Polycystic Ovary Syndrome (PCOS)

In today's world, up to fifteen percent of women have PCOS. PCOS is diagnosed when at least two of the following symptoms are present:[3]

- Anovulation (no ovulating, so no period)
- Elevated levels of blood serum androgens
- Hyperandrogenism (such as extra facial hair, acne, and patchy hair, called androgenic alopecia)
- Polycystic ovaries are found in an ultrasound

PCOS develops usually in teens. It starts as irregular periods and later presents as infertility, hyperandrogenism. Later in life, PCOS contributes to obesity and cardiac disorders such as syndrome X and/or Z, diabetes, and high blood pressure.

PCOS is on the rise.

OSA statistically is much higher in those who have PCOS, listed at twenty-two percent in one study in comparison to two to five percent of adult women who do not have PCOS. Women with PCOS were more likely than their teenage counterparts with PCOS to have sleep apnea.[3]

Menopause: Women are more likely to develop sleep disordered breathing in menopause. The risk of developing sleep issues doubles after menopause. The most common age to be diagnosed with sleep-disordered breathing is sixty-five years in women, whereas it is fifty-five years old in men. There is less natural drive from the brain stem to drive respiration. Women in menopause generally gain weight, which also contributes to sleep troubles. In women, there is a linear progression of likelihood to suffer sleep issues as age increases.[1]

In summary, women's hormones create a different effect on their breathing anatomy, and this is can be the case when there is a low AHI score on a sleep study but where the woman has at least a partial airway obstruction. In these cases, treating for sleep issues is just as important as in the man who has a high AHI score. Even mild OSA scores based upon a low AHI reading in a sleep study can be comparable and treated with equal concerns as a man with a high AHI score. AHI scores were explained in Chapter 3.

Men's Hormones and Sleep

Testosterone, the male hormone, functions on a circadian rhythm of its own. It peaks during sleep and has its lowest level in late afternoon. It works in tandem with another sort of rhythm of luteinizing hormone every ninety minutes. Sleep increases testosterone in the body. When low testosterone is present, these disorders can present:[5]

- Poor sleep quality
- Less duration of sleep
- Circadian rhythm disorders
- Sleep breathing disorders

OSA does not have a direct effect on testosterone levels, but because OSA contributes to obesity, it can indirectly affect testosterone levels.

Not getting enough sleep (sleep deprivation) will lead to lower testosterone levels in men. This effect is worsened as a man ages. So, a younger man is able to recover his testosterone levels quicker, and his levels never drop as much as is likely in an older man.

A man who suffers from the symptoms listed above should consider having his testosterone levels checked.

Macuna pruriens, the Ayruvedic herb mentioned earlier, is linked to increasing testosterone. It also can lower prolactin in women who are suffering from adrenal fatigue. Macuna brings back hormonal balance and boosts natural transmitters needed for sleep like dopamine.[5]

Erectile dysfunction in men is associated with oral sleep apnea, and it seems to have to do with the nitric oxide pathway. CPAP has been studied and found to help E.D., but oral devices have not yet been studied for E.D.[6]

In summary, obese women and men with sleep disturbances will benefit from losing weight through diet and exercise along with treatment for sleep to heal and live their best life.[3]

Thyroid Function and Sleep

An underactive and/or an overactive thyroid gland will affect your sleep. Knowing if your thyroid is functioning in a proper range by producing thyroid hormones is another step towards ensuring your best night's rest. The normal range for TSH (thyroid stimulating hormone) is between 0.5 mU/l and 5.0 mU/l. A high TSH is generally an indication that you have an underactive thyroid (hypothyroidism) and an abnormally low TSH indicates you may be hyperthyroid (Graves' disease).

Forty percent of patients with underactive thyroid or Hashimoto's disease also have sleep apnea. Sometimes sleep apnea causes the thyroid issue, and sometimes the thyroid issue contributes to a patient developing sleep disordered breathing (an AHI score over 5). In these patients, sometimes the sleep disordered breathing condition has been reversed when the patient takes a prescription for thyroxine. The way that the thyroid medication works to help reduce the sleep disorder is that the swelling of the tissue in the airway is reduced as the thyroid begins to function more normally.[8]

One way of treatment does not suit all patients. A study was published on "Is thyroid testing necessary in all patients who have sleep apnea?" And the answer seems to be that this is only recommended in patients who are in the highest risk group for underactive thyroid (over the age of sixty years).[9]

The main links between sleep issues and an overactive thyroid (Graves' disease) include:

1. Occurrences of night sweats
2. Difficulty falling asleep
3. Less REM sleep (because of night sweats and falling asleep later and getting up at the same time in the morning)

Let's examine some of the additional factors that influence thyroid function by looking at what chemical cocktail the thyroid requires to function. Healthy thyroid, breast, ovarian and uterine and prostate tissue (all of these listed except thyroid are considered male and female gonad tissue) function happen when the body receives a proper supply of iodine. In today's American diet, most of us do not receive as much iodine as we need.

If you wonder how well your thyroid is functioning, a blood test can reveal where you are. Blood levels of thyroid hormones are used to diagnose an over or an under thyroid, and these levels have changed in the last twenty years. Here are current lab levels of various thyroid hormones:

Lab number	Optimal Range
Free T4	1.1 ng/dL
Free T3	Greater than 3.2 pg/mL
Reverse T3	Less than a 10:1 ration of RT3 to FT3
TSH	1.0-2.0 IU/mL or lower; Pregnant women less than 2.5 IU/mL
Thyroid peroxidase antibodies	Less than 9 IU/ mL or negative
Thyroglobulin antibodies	Less than 4 IU/mL or negative

Thyroid and Iodine

The thyroid gland needs iodine to function properly. Here are some interesting statistics about the state of Americans' Health and their need for iodine:

- At least one third of women over the age of forty take thyroid medications for either overactive or for underactive thyroid function.
- One in three men develop prostate cancer, and this cancer rate is increasing.
- PCOS (polycystic ovarian syndrome) is on the rise.
- Hypothyroidism is on the rise.
- Recommended daily intake of iodine is 150 micrograms iodine daily, 220 micrograms in pregnancy.

Your thyroid gland is located in your neck. It absorbs iodine and the amino acid tyrosine to make hormones, especially thyroxine (T4) and triiodothyronine (T3), The thyroid gland affects:

- Breathing and heart rate,
- The central nervous system
- Body weight, muscle strength
- Menstrual cycles: frequency and heaviness
- Body temperature regulation

Classic signs of underactive thyroid can include:

- Slow heart rate and constipation/weight gain
- Trouble sleeping
- Fatigue
- Difficulty concentrating, depression
- Dry skin, hair
- Sensitivity to cold
- Frequent, heavy periods
- Joint and muscle pain

Classic signs of an overactive thyroid can include:

- Rapid heart rate and diarrhea/weight loss
- Anxiety, irritability, hyperactivity
- Sweating or sensitivity to high temperatures, shaking, hair loss
- Light or missed menstrual periods

Breast Cancer and Low Thyroid Diagnosis

There seem to be connections with various types of cancer and thyroid issues. Much research has centered around breast cancer risk and thyroid disease. There does seem to be an association between these tissues that concentrate iodine and cancer. While we do not fully understand the mechanism of this risk, we do know that when there are either overactive or underactive thyroid issues, breast cancer risk increases.[11] Another study indicated a significant association between thyroid autoantibody levels and thyroid gland issues, particularly nontoxic goiters, and breast cancer. In dentistry, a sign of an underactive thyroid is a swollen tongue. Dentists have occasionally been reported to be the first identifier of a thyroid issue in a patient based upon this clinical finding of an enlarged tongue.[1]

Being low in iodine causes TSH to be released, potentially rendering a patient the diagnosis of underactive thyroid. The underactive thyroid is treated with thyroid medication, but the underlying cause of diagnosis, low iodine, is never addressed in this scenario. Thus, tissue needing iodine never receives it, leading to disease. So when getting a diagnosis for thyroid function, please make sure you have had your iodine levels checked.

An inexpensive at-home test you can manage yourself to indicate iodine insufficiency is to purchase some liquid iodine drops, such as Lugol's brand. Paint the inside of your arm, opposite your elbow. It is said that if you are low in iodine, the yellow stain left behind from the Lugol's will disappear before 24 hours (assuming you have not washed the skin here). Verify iodine levels with your doctor through a special blood test.

If low in iodine levels, you might consider taking iodine supplements along with or before beginning thyroid supplementation. If you already take thyroid medication, it is still helpful to know if you are low in iodine so that you can rectify this problem, thereby lowering your risk of breast cancer.

Breast, Ovarian, and Prostate Tissue and Iodine

The breast, ovary, and prostate tissue also need iodine, so supplementing when low protects all of these organs from developing cancer or undesirable changes. Lumpy breasts and ovarian cysts are signs of non-health in these tissues, and frequently iodine supplementation can improve these conditions. Prostate or uterine cancer seems to also be prevented with adequate iodine intake.

Halide chemical elements including fluorine, bromine, and chlorine compete on cells for the same spots as iodine, which is also a halide chemical (meaning these all behave and are attracted chemically to the same places in the body). Halide chemicals are increasingly found in a variety of places in our modern environment. Bromine is added to fertilizers, so even organic produce may contain this chemical. It is also found in many bread and pastry products. Fluorine is also called fluoride in particular forms, and it is found in the water of canned foods, manufactured drinks, slurry-formed foods such as cereals, and in our municipal water supplies. It is also a byproduct of the fertilizer industry. With so many sources of fluoride in today's environment, this is why fluoride is not as necessary in today's world for cavity prevention in the teeth. Chlorine, like fluoride, is added to municipal water supplies and in swimming pools to disinfect. Halide chemical exposure is so commonplace in today's society, so your effort to increase your intake of iodine from foods and possibly supplements can be excellent for disease prevention. Even folks ingesting regular supplies of iodine could end up with the risk of the wrong chemical competing and getting mistakenly taken up by a cell as needed iodine because other chemicals can behave like iodine. Iodine supplementation can help prevent this from occurring.

Remember iodized salt? We began adding iodine to salt back in the 1940's. With the advent of cooking with natural sea salt, many of us Americans have cut out what had become our main source of iodine in our modern diet. Good natural sources of iodine today include sea vegetables and fish. Perhaps some will consider using iodized salt again. Others might take iodine drops such as Lugol's brand.

I have seen many, many dental patients who suffer with ailments of breast, uterine, prostate thyroid; potentially many are low on iodine. When the problems are so common and the solutions could be simple for major disease prevention, it behooves me to put good information out to the general public.

Case Study: Terry the Thyroid Patient Who Can't Sleep

Terry came in to see me for a checkup. She had been a regular patient of mine for about fifteen years. She seemed different this time and had a lot going on personally. She reported that after her forty-seventh birthday, she began to suspect that she suffers from an underactive thyroid. She wanted to see if she could make a difference with her diet before she goes back to her doctor to get tested and try a medication. She was very tired, and her mother had recently passed away. She had been biting her tongue and injured herself a number of times because it just seemed to be in the way of her teeth. She admitted that she was grinding her teeth at night. She was also trying to lose weight. Springtime was in the air, and she lamented that she had some swelling around her forearms that she hoped she could eliminate by lifting weights.

My Recommendation for Terry

1. I told her that she needed to follow up with her doctor to have a thyroid function blood test. Meanwhile, I recommended she try some at-home techniques which may shed some light on

her condition. The swelling of her upper arms (confirmed by pinching the flesh here) left an indentation in the skin, indicating myxedema. This is classic for a low-functioning thyroid symptom.

2. We did a skin patch test with Lugol's drops, and the skin patch had disappeared within six hours. Terry called us after her appointment to let us know. Sometimes, we do a patch test at the office so the patient can learn more about themselves. It is up to the patient to seek medical care after the dental appointment. Remember, it was suggested that Terry was hypothyroid (low thyroid) because the yellow stain from the drops had disappeared within twenty-four hours (often happens in a couple hours with a low thyroid patient). I told Terry to follow up with a doctor in a month and that she could try self-dosing with a dropperful of 2% Lugol's drops in a gallon of water daily.

3. I told Terry about using filtered water. Most water filters and bottled water companies do not have filter for fluoride. Fluoride could potentially compete with iodine on the iodine receptors on the cell membranes in her body because it is also a halide chemical. All halide chemicals are in the same family of chemicals in the Periodic Table of Elements, and this family includes iodine, fluorine, chlorine, and bromine. Your body must have iodine to be healthy. That is why you see iodine in the US RDA (suggested does 150 micrograms/daily which was raised in 2018 from 120 micrograms daily) whereas you will not see a recommended daily dose of bromine, chorine, or fluorine (or their derivatives). Because of the increasing amounts of these other halides in the environment that compete with iodine in your body, supplementing has become increasingly more important. You can consider improving the water quality at her home with a reverse osmosis water filter. If removing fluoride from water is

important to you, then you need to buy a separate filter for the system specifically for fluoride. See the resources page at the end of this book for suggestions on vendors.

4. I suggested Terry eat more sea vegetables (kelp salt crystals) and use iodized salt (takes about a quarter teaspoon of iodized salt for your daily iodine intake), seaweed, and eggs. Five dried prunes daily will give Terry about 9% of her daily suggested iodine dose and are a vegetarian option, and one cup cooked lima beans will give her about 10%. Also, I mentioned to Terry that wild caught white fish (such as cod and tuna) and shrimp, while being a source of iodine, should probably not be ingested more often than about twice weekly due to the mercury content in these food sources. Some fish are more laden with heavy metals than others (often bottom feeders).

5. I told Terry I recommended supplementing with 600 micrograms of selenium daily. Selenium can also be obtained by eating several Brazil nuts daily. Macadamia and hazelnuts also contain selenium. Selenium helps iodine absorption. Selenium is an essential mineral, and it's not typically measured in routine blood tests.

6. I suggested Terry try the Hypothyroidism diet. Generally, the Hypothyroidism diet is a good way to keep your thyroid functioning at its best when you are faced with low thyroid. With this diet, you basically eat whole foods and reduce consumption of Brussels sprouts, cabbage, cauliflower, kale, bok choy, and turnip greens because these foods can reduce the thyroid glands ability to absorb iodine.

7. Terry had been fatigued, and we suspected her thyroid was functioning at a lower than optimal level. This could affect her sleep. Terry's tongue was very swollen and had scalloped edges suggesting hypoactive thyroid. Terry visited her physician

to confirm the diagnosis by measuring her thyroid hormone levels. Terry began taking Thyroxine to help get her thyroid gland functioning more normally. As Terry regained better thyroid function, she did experience increased energy and less daytime sleepiness. Her tongue became less swollen, and she had not bit it in a long while when we last saw her. Because she was sleeping well and feeling much better, she postponed a sleep test at this time. We might have had Terry come in for an airway scan if she had not gotten better. Sometimes, patients who have an anatomically small airway experience low thyroid symptoms that can be addressed with an oral sleep appliance that can remodel the airway. See the chapter on Airway Size Matters for more information.

Notice that these suggestions do not go outside the range of treating dental disease. These suggestions involve follow-up with a medical doctor and how to incorporate more iodine in the diet at home. Hopefully, the dental professional can also assist Terry with selecting a doctor that would be well-matched to understand Terry and her concerns.

Stress Hormones and Sleep

The stress response system of the human body is made up of several components of the central nervous system. These include:

- Neurons that release corticotropin release hormone in the hypothalamic paraventricular nucleus
- Nuclei of the brain stem and surrounding helper centers called the hypothalamicpituitaryadrenal (HPA) axis and the peripheral autonomic nervous system.

The main function of these components is to maintain a balance, called homeostasis, in resting states and when the body faces a stress.

Stress and stress hormones influence how much, how long, and how well you sleep. Here are some statistics:[13]

- Deep sleep has a slowing effect on the HPA axis.
- A patient who is given glucocorticoids or who has an activation of the HPA axis can experience sleeplessness.
- Insomnia is associated with a twenty-four-hour increase of ACTH and cortisol secretion.
- When there is excessive daytime sleepiness, there is an increase in pro inflammatory cytokines interleukin 6 (IL6) and/or tumor necrosis factor (TNF). These same chemicals are activated with many of the inflammatory conditions discussed in the last chapter, sometimes even periodontal disease. Daytime sleepiness is caused from troubles like sleep apnea, narcolepsy, and idiopathic hypersomnia.
- Sleep deprivation leads to sleepiness and daytime hypersecretion of IL-6. When sleep is disrupted, more cortisol (stress hormone) is released into the blood stream. Overall, individuals getting regular poor sleep have higher circulating cortisol than their counterparts.
- On average, cortisol levels are higher in those getting shorter than average sleep time.[14]

**

The figure below illustrates the relationship between parts of the nervous system that regulate stress and sleep states and REM sleep. A solid line represents promotion/stimulation; a dotted line represents inhibition or interruption.[14,15,16]

CRH = corticotropicreleasing hormone

ACTH = corticotropin

LC/NE = sympathetic nervous system/epinephrine/adrenaline producer

AVP = arginine metabolic pathway (makes Nitric Oxide before age forty years)

GH = growth hormone

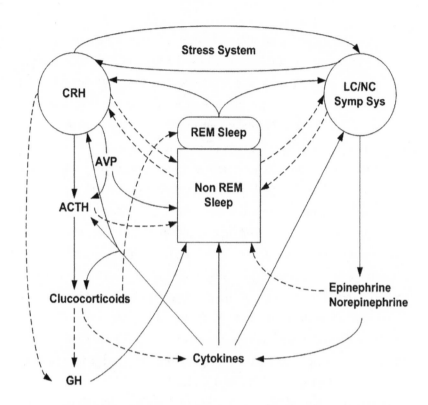

Higher amounts of REM sleep are associated with higher activation of the HPA axis. REM sleep increases in patients who have melancholic depression.

In a physically or emotionally stressful situation, the paraventricular nucleus of the brain releases corticotropic releasing hormone (CRH). Then two chemicals are released in the stress response cascade:

1. Increased adrenocorticotropin hormone (ACTH) is released by the pituitary gland of the brain, and

2. Cortisol is released from the adrenal glands, which are located on top of the kidney. Cortisol not only is released in a stressful situation, but it also helps us to regulate how we use our nutrients from protein, carbohydrates, and fats in our diet. It also helps us to maintain blood pressure and controls inflammation.

There is a sleep-rousing effect of CRH in adults. Children seem less sensitive to the release of CRH. In adults, the result of CRH has an effect of less time spent sleeping and less slow-wave sleep. When ACTH is released, there is an activation of the nervous system. We sleep less time, less deeply, and get less REM sleep when ACTH is higher than normal. We are still discovering the effects of the stress reactions of the nervous system in people who start with poor sleep and many more studies will have to be conducted to understand poor sleep on the CRH and ACTH axis system. In rats, we know that in a state of sleep deprivation, the rat responds with a stress response of having higher ACTH and corticosteroid levels and increased epinephrine circulating in the blood stream. What is currently believed is that people with insomnia will generally have higher cortisol levels in the blood, and these people have higher rates of Type II diabetes, poor mental focus, and higher rates of hypertension.

Antidepressants can suppress the activity of the HPA axis[15] and therefore they may help with a patient to get more sleep and reduce cortisol levels even in someone without depression.[16]

One study showed that a CPAP machine used for only three months in obese patients with sleep apnea could help regulate the stress system and that by eliminating intermittent hypoxia episodes, the stress response was normalized in the patients. Hypertension was reduced in obese men in this study.[17,18] Short-term use of a CPAP had significant effects on cortisol levels in those studied.

When the HPA axis is impaired, there is more activity with the growth hormone axis.

Glucocorticoids Suppress REM Sleep[19]

It seems that some cortisol is needed for REM sleep, but excess cortisol inhibits REM sleep, possibly by suppressing CRH.

What happens if your adrenal glands either under produce or over-produce their hormones, and how does this potentially affect sleep?

Addison's Disease

Adrenal gland insufficiency is called Addison's disease, and it is a type of autoimmune disease in which the body is not making enough natural cortisol or aldosterone. We have covered what cortisol's function is but not aldosterone. Aldosterone's function in the body it to help the kidneys regulate the amount of salt and water in the body, which means it has an effect on blood pressure and blood volume. John F. Kennedy suffered from Addison's disease. People suffering from Addison's disease generally have chronic fatigue, among other problems. Patients with untreated Addison's disease have more incidence of sleep fragmentation, delayed REM onset, and overall decreased REM sleep. These changes can often be reversed with treatment using doses of hydrocortisone, so it is thought that REM sleep may need cortisol secretion.

Adrenal Failure[30,31]

I have had so many patients come in with diagnosis of adrenal failure. What is this condition? Adrenal failure is marked by at least some of these symptoms:

- Extreme fatigue and history of life stress(es)
- Weight loss and decreased appetite
- Darkening of the skin
- Low blood pressure, feeling faint
- Cravings for salt
- Abdominal pain
- Tummy problems, including nausea, diarrhea and/or vomiting
- Depression
- Hair loss or sexual dysfunction in women
- Achy joints

Causes of adrenal failure are stress-related and can mimic a mild form of Addison's disease.

Cushing Syndrome[27,32]

Cushing syndrome is a condition caused from a pituitary gland tumor that creates overstimulation of the adrenal glands. Sometimes symptoms of Cushing syndrome can develop as a result of using medications such as prednisone. Symptoms include:

- Obesity
- Acne
- High blood pressure
- Red stretch marks
- In women, more hair and irregular periods

Your body chemistry changes when you develop obesity. When you are obese, chemicals are released into the blood stream that create a cascade of effects including increased risk of sleep apnea. In one study, thirty-two percent of patients with Cushing syndrome had at least mild sleep apnea and eighteen percent had moderate to severe sleep apnea (AHI over 17.5 per hour).[20] These patients were not noted to be obese or have other physical changes sometimes associated with Cushing syndrome (changes in the skull bones). They seemed normal in physical appearance.

When we are sick, there can be an introduction of cytokines as an immune response. Cytokines interact with the HPA axis and there is an increased need for sleep for the immune system to fight the illness. The cytokine IL-1 has been shown to create more slow-wave activity, to create the body's need to increase sleep. IL-1 has been linked to the onset of slow-wave sleep.[21]

Decreased amounts of IL-6 secretion have been linked to better sleep. In another study, IL-6 was administered and found to cause the need for much more sleep and contributed to feelings of great fatigue.[22,23,28]

In another study, IL-6 and cortisol levels were found to be higher in older versus younger adults, which suggests that these chemicals may rise some in the aging process. IL-6 is associated with sleep/wake cycles, and cortisol is associated with REM sleep.[22,23,28]

It has also been found that TNF (tumor necrosis factor) also creates a need for more sleep in the body.[23,24,25,29,30]

Studies show that the peak time of chemicals in the blood stream is altered in people with daytime sleepiness in comparison to those who report sleeping well.

Aging seems to be associated with increased wear and tear on the HPA axis. "Rode hard and put up wet" comes to mind here. A life filled with stress that has activated the HPA axis will create a very active HPA axis and contribute to aging. Increased levels of IL-1 and IL-6 will enhance this effect.

In summary: hormones involved in the human stress response alter sleep patterns, amount of sleep, and types of sleep. These hormones are also connected to the release of cytokines, or inflammatory chemicals that contribute towards diseases processes. Being in touch with your body's response to stressors in your life will be helpful to your ability to maintain wellness, to age slower, and to sleep.

The Adrenal Failure Case: Dr. Randy

Adrenal failure is often the result of a high-stress lifestyle. This affects both men and women. Adrenal glands sit on top of the kidneys in a patient's abdomen. Adrenal failure refers to the health situation occurring when the adrenal gland hormones are not properly functioning. There can be too little hormone being released from the adrenal gland or too much.

Clues that a patient may be suffering from adrenal failure are incredible fatigue following illness or a stressful event in their life, a feeling of emotional burnout, sugar and salt cravings, increasing reliance on stimulants like caffeine, and some digestive problems tending towards IBS (irritable bowel syndrome). When you consider that about twenty percent of patients have IBS symptoms that may not have a proper diagnosis, it begs one to consider if adrenal failure could be a player. One does not have to present with all of these symptoms to be suffering from adrenal failure. Some individuals also have hypoglycemic episodes (low blood sugar), darkening of skin (hyperpigmentation), low blood pressure, and/ or history of fainting spells.

Treatment recommendations: Again, I recommend seeking a doctor to assist in diagnosing and treating, but the dental team should be a support for the patient. We can recommend gentle guidance for this patient who is becoming desperate to feel better. Just as adrenal failure does not just suddenly happen, it is a road spiraling downward and a climb upwards that takes typically a number of months to achieve health and energy again. The patient is ready to start with gentle!

Dr. Randy: a thirty-nine-year-old physician came to see me for a checkup. He had contracted bronchitis in the summer months. His asthma had acted up after his family moved into a new-construction house with continued construction going on all around their homestead. Randy had the stress of a new mortgage and the needs of two young children changing schools and a marriage to handle while seeing patients fulltime daily. Physician burnout is a real issue in our country. Please listen to your friends and family, patients and colleagues who are tired working as caregivers. Randy was a vegetarian – had been one for years. He enjoyed a nightly glass of wine or two. Besides wanting a dental checkup, his chief complaint to me was about his fatigue.

Recommendations

Anti-inflammatory diet: Eat whole food – fruits and vegetables – but consider adding either fish oil (or try vegan omega-3 supplements) to lift mood (buy higher EPA to DHA fatty acid content). Omega-3s are wonderful for turning down many inflammatory pathways. Reduce alcohol consumption to once weekly while battling this fatigue.

DGL supplements: Deglycyrrhizinated licorice supplements. Derived from licorice (the herb, not the candy), these flavored (sometimes

German chocolate) are a tasty (sweet) way to help rebuild your adrenal glands. Licorice is an adaptogenic herb and also helps with mucous to coat the GI (digestive track). People with high blood pressure generally stay away from licorice because of its potential effects on blood pressure. Licorice, the herb, has been documented as being used for centuries for digestive problems and fatigue.

Adrenal herbal formula or a combination of herbal supplements: Consider a supplement combination either commercially produced or formulated by a local herbalist to approach improving adrenal fatigue with gentleness. Generally popular herbs used include: rhodiola and Siberian ginseng (also called eleuthero) for daytime formulas and ashwagandha or holy basil for nighttime formulas. For dosages for this herb and all others mentioned, please consult the table in the Tables section of this book.

Rhodiola: The Vikings were known to have on their cruises and is attributed with contributing to the legendary strength and fortitude the Vikings. Alone, it may be a little strong. It is available over the counter as a tincture or as a capsule.

Siberian Ginseng, or eleuthero: This is quite different from its cousins in the plant world, Asian and American ginsengs. Eleuthero is known for a gentler adaptogenic "get up and go" effect on the body than rhodiola. Again, it has been used for centuries throughout Eurasia for its healing properties.

Holy Basil: It's similar in its cortisol effect as ashwagandha. Traditionally, holy basil (a different variety of basil than your typical garden-variety basil) was used by yogis in a tea (leaves not traditionally eaten) to help them reach a higher meditative state. This adaptogenic herb is also rejuvenating to the adrenal glands. This is available as a capsule or as Tulsi tea.

Vitamin B complex: Usually I recommend a formula containing methylated B12 and methylated folate (methylated folic acid or vitamin

B9). Possibly as much as fifty percent of our population has a recessive gene SNP (called SNIP) that creates inefficiency in methylating (or adding a CH3 group to vitamin B12 and to folic acid) that enables absorption. Individuals with MTHFR gene often suffer from low levels of B12 and B9. These 2 vitamins help for coping with stress. Enhancing stores of B12 and B9 help alleviate MTHFR as a contributing factor to the fatigue in patients who may have adrenal failure. Dr. Randy was also recommended for B12 testing to make sure he was not low in B12 or iron.

More rest! This is maybe common sense, but sometimes people need to hear that they need to rest more. Some people have a hard time giving themselves permission to take care of themselves first before others. I also tell people to select one thing daily (at least) that will bring them joy to do as a daily activity. By the way, a few months later, Dr. Randy tested positive with a polysomnograph for severe sleep apnea.

Dr. Randy wore a CPAP for about six months which helped him to sleep easier while he got used to his oral sleep apnea device, a Vivos appliance which will be discussed in a later chapter. He started losing some weight during this time without trying, and we both thought it was due to his ability to sleep easier with the CPAP.

These nights, Dr. Randy is wearing his Vivos appliance, an Oral DNA, in lieu of the CPAP for his condition. His device will allow him to grow his breathing airway over time which will help him to rest much better as one of the causes of his ongoing health issues (his compromised airway) will be eased. He has also created a sleep routine.

Chapter 8:

Stress, Lifestyle Choices, and Their Consequences on Sleep

"A mother's arms are made of tenderness,
and children sleep soundly in them."
– Victor Hugo

I n Today's world, the integrative-minded dental team can transcend the roles of traditional dentistry and be a resource for whole body care for patients. This is proactive and very helpful in today's medical environment when many do not have consistent care with the same providers year after year.

The dental office can screen patients for mind, body, and spiritual health. They can take note of pharmaceutical drugs taken regularly by the patient and caution the patient about vitamin depletion made more likely by such drugs. The dental team can listen to family tendencies or the perceived life struggles of the patient because we know the family history. Plus, the dental team can refer patients to the other practitioners in their area who can help patients in their healing journey. Here, I am talking about the team knowing who the best acupuncturist, counselor, therapeutic touch/reiki/spiritual healer is in town.

***

Adverse Childhood Experiences (ACE) and Sleep

Did you know that Adverse Childhood Experiences (ACE) can really warp your ability to sleep and therefore to heal?

For those who have had ACE, there are implications about who will be more likely to become stricken from chronic disease including: ischemic heart disease, cancer, chronic pulmonary disease, emphysema (COPD), liver disease, and tendency for skeletal fractures.

In a 1998 study, it was shown that there was a statistical correlation between all of the above chronic health problems and the number of ACE.[1]

Below is the typical ACE Questionnaire.[1] The higher the number of ACE's you have experienced, the more likely you are to experience chronic health issues later in life.

Do you know if you have had any adverse childhood experiences?

ACE Questionnaire

Answer appropriately if the question applies to your childhood exposure. Give yourself one point for each line where your answer is yes.

Abuse by category:

Psychological

(Did a parent or other adult in the household...)

- Often or very often swear at, insult, or put you down?
- Often or very often act in a way that made you afraid that you would be physically hurt?

Physical

(Did a parent or other adult in the household...)

- Often or very often push, grab, shove, or slap you?
- Often or very often hit you so hard that you had marks or were injured?

Sexual

(Did an adult or person at least five years older ever...)

- Touch or fondle you in a sexual way?
- Have you touch their body in a sexual way?
- Attempt oral, anal, or vaginal intercourse with you?
- Actually have oral, anal, or vaginal intercourse with you?

Household Dysfunction By Category

- Substance abuse
- Live with someone who was a problem drinker or alcoholic?
- Live with anyone who used street drugs?
- Mental abuse
- Was a household member depressed or mentally ill?
- Did a household member attempt suicide?
- Mother treated violently
- Was your mother (or stepmother) sometimes, often, or very often pushed, grabbed, slapped, or had something thrown at her?
- Sometimes, often, or very often kicked, bitten, hit with a fist, or hit with something hard?
- Ever repeatedly hit over at least a few minutes?
- Ever threatened with, or hurt by, a knife or gun?

- Criminal behavior in household
- Did a household member go to prison?

*An exposure to one or more items listed under the set of questions for each category.

Because of the startling findings of the ACE study, another study was devised that assessed sleep disturbances in adults and a connection to ACE. The findings reflected that thirty-three percent of those who had experienced ACE had trouble falling or staying asleep and that twenty-four percent of those studied had daytime sleepiness. Compared with individuals who reported an ACE score of 0, people having an ACE score were over twice as likely to report trouble falling or staying asleep and twice as likely to feel daytime sleepiness after a good night's sleep. The number of ACE's reported by the questionnaire was found to be proportional to the sleep disturbances.[2]

In another study in adolescents, it was found that in maltreated adolescent females who had post-traumatic stress disorders, it was necessary to treat mental health symptoms while addressing physical causes of sleep disturbances for the girls to heal physically and mentally and to ultimately sleep better. These teenage girls had both depression and PTSD symptoms. In general, it was also found that maltreated teens required more sleep than their non-abused counterparts.[3]

It stands to reason that it may be possible that having an ACE may impact how you as an adult may approach taking care of yourself. You may wait longer before booking an appointment for yourself when a health concern is identified. To know that you may have been a victim of ACE may give you courage to take a step forward and care for yourself sooner than before.

To manage stress, consider the power of positive thinking, exercise, therapy, self-compassion, love in your life from yourself and your inner circle of family and friends. Incorporate more of the love part into your life to feel better.

Also, I hope you will consider the importance of reducing stress in your household and in minimizing creating childhood trauma as you are parenting!

Electromagnetic Field (EMF) and Sleep

EMF is an abbreviation for electromagnetic field. It also needs to be considered in how it affects the quality of your sleep. Long-term exposure to EMF is a reality in our modern lives. We use EMF for internet anything and for cell phone use. Imagine our lives without EMF today! We are also increasing our exposure to EMF by adding 5G to communities all over the globe using satellite technology. One of the concerns some have about EMF has to do with the many unrecognized health implications of using EMF. We do not have the ability to see into the future with regard to the true fallout of what we will be able to see in fifty more years' time.

We know that large exposures to EMF can cause instantaneous death as has occurred on U.S. Navy ships.

So what is known about EMF and sleep? In a study by Graham and Cook, it was learned that an intermittent exposure to a magnetic field during sleep time will disrupt sleep.[4] We also know that this has greater health implications when it happens during sleep times than during waking times because of the healing process that should occur at night.[5] In a study in Iran on workers living in high voltage electrical environments, a definite correlation was made between amounts of EMF exposure and poor sleep. Poor sleep in this study was defined by how long it took to fall asleep, how long one slept, how rested one felt after sleep, and if one woke some during sleep.[6]

For those who consider themselves to be sensitive to EMF, exposure has also been linked to headaches, nervousness, general fatigue, and leads to difficulty concentrating on tasks.[7]

So how can you limit your exposure to EMF while sleeping?

First, it is essential to know what your exposure may be. Determine how far your sleeping quarters are to your internet router, cell phone, computer, and Roku movie equipment. Consider purchasing a meter that measures EMF. These cost around a hundred dollars and can be purchased on the internet from companies such as LessEMF.com.

If you find you have a lot of EMF near your sleeping quarters, consider how you can change this influence in your sleep situation. Perhaps you move your router or turn it off at night. Keep your cell phone and computer away from your bed. Some purchase canopies or other fabric to use as shielding from EMF that is unavoidable. I have found that many hotels have the router located inside the nightstand of the hotel room; one could consider wearing a fabric shield or using a shielding blanket for protection.

Lifestyle Choices and Sleep

What basic sleep routine choices can you incorporate tonight for yourself and family so everyone sleeps better?

Practice what I call the Dynamics of Sleep hygiene, just like your mom might have done for you when you were a baby! This is self-care for sleeping! Develop a schedule and routine for sleep. Just as you might schedule for a young child who is getting ready to start the school year, begin prioritizing your own bedtime.

Keep your bedtime the same on weeknights as on weekends.

Limit your exposure to blue light at least two hours before bedtime. There are some (mostly) inexpensive products on the market that can help normalize light and help relax your body to prepare you for your best sleep. We have discussed the six-dollar magnesium supplement and EMF fabric shielding or turning off EMF around your bed as choices.

Lighting in your room makes a difference in getting you into a time-to-go-to-sleep mood. Blue wavelength light from TV's, computers, or cell phones is energizing. Orange glasses (available for purchase on the internet) block the blue wavelength without disrupting your ability to discern text or obstruct viewing a good movie. These look like sunglasses and cost around thirty dollars. You can also adjust the lighting in your bedroom with dimmer switches.

Consider taping your mouth if you mouth breathe. Mouth tape or medical adhesive tape can be used if you are noticing that either you or a loved one tends to sleep with their mouth open. Mouth breathing needs to be corrected as it does not allow the body to maintain a proper ratio of oxygen: carbon dioxide to nitric oxide. Try taping the mouth during waking hours first so you do not fell panicky when taping before bed. Practice Buteyko breathing a full several minutes before placing the tape to help open up nasal passages. If you have strong allergies or a cold, do not try mouth taping until these health issues have resolved themselves because it will make success more difficult. Patrick McKeown's book *Close Your Mouth* is an excellent resource on this topic. Also consider looking up Buteyko breathing on the internet for videos or more information.

Consider trying Breathe-Rite strips, available over the counter, to see if these help you sleep as a temporary measure.

There is something available to everyone, all the time: the Emotional Freedom Technique (EMF). A similar treatment is called Havening Technique. EMF has been extensively studied and found to calm people who find themselves in all types of stressful situations, from dental work to bumpy airline flights. EMF involves deep breathing, inhalation, and exhalation through the nose while squeezing acupressure points that ease anxiety. All the while, you're thinking about a positive outcome to the current stressor.

To practice EMF:

1. Get your mind straight: imagine completing and congratulating yourself on completing your current difficulty.

2. Breathe. If you are doing this correctly, your tummy will expand below your diaphragm first and the filling of lungs extends then upwards to your shoulders upon inhalation (but your shoulders will not rise). Hold your breath for a few seconds, then begin to slowly exhale. Some healthcare practitioners call this type of breathing deep the 4-7-8-method, meaning take four seconds to inhale, hold for seven, then exhale for eight seconds. The slow, regulated breathing decreases your heart rate and promotes up-regulation of the parasympathetic nervous system. This type of breathing also decreases use of accessory muscles (cranial nerve XI) in assisting you to breathe. In other words, your breathing is actually easier for your body to achieve.

3. The technique involves activating or squeezing with your fingers various acupressure points as pictured below to reduce anxiety (hold at least ten seconds):[9]

Picture of acupressure points for EMF

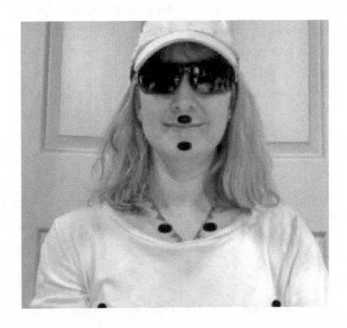

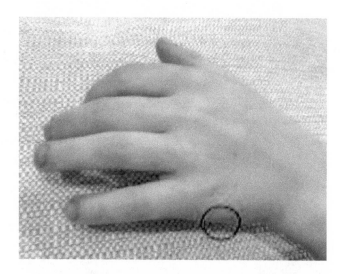

1. There are also some good videos on YouTube for a self-taught course on EMF. Children's Hospital of Minnesota routinely is teaching EMF to the patients to reduce fear of procedures. EMF has been shown in medical research to help people suffering from chronic pain, depression, anxiety, and post-traumatic stress disorder (PTSD).[8]

2. Emotional Freedom Technique has been found to help relieve symptoms of PTSD (post-traumatic stress disorder), chronic pain, anxiety, phobias, and depression. EMF has been shown to relieve or downgrade the sympathetic nervous system and therefore improve health.

3. Do not have more than two alcoholic beverages (preferably drink no alcohol less than four or five hours before bedtime).

4. When we metabolize alcohol, it can rouse us from deeper sleep about six hours after we consume it. If this falls into the window of time when you are trying to hit REM sleep, you will inevitably not be able to get the REM sleep your body craves.

5. Consider supplements, essential oils such as lavender, or herbal teas to help induce and maintain sleep.

6. Get sleep tested by your doctor or dentist to understand why you don't sleep! The advantage of getting tested at the dental office is that you may be more likely to hear about oral appliances from your dentist than from your doctor. The dentist will have to corroborate with your doctor on the diagnosis, but this way you will have more than one set of eyes on your treatment plan solution suited best for you.

7. If you are found to have an anatomical reason for sleeping poorly, then determine what fits you best to solve your issue. This discovery and information gathering process is the main purpose of this book. If you have a problem, should you:

   a. Consider surgery for sleep apnea in terms of either having an implant to stimulate breathing or a tonsillectomy/adenoidectomy or a uvulectomy?

   b. Consider wearing a CPAP?

   c. Consider wearing an oral appliance to correct your sleep issue?

Which option – A, B, or C – above is best for you?

Chapter 9:

Size Matters in Airway and Sleep

"Sleep is that golden chain that ties
health and our bodies together."
– Thomas Dekker

I t's time to take a look at sleep solutions through surgical and/or through appliance therapy. The bottom line: If you have a large open airway, sleep will be more easily achievable.

Personally, I prefer non-surgical therapies to address sleep issues. Nowadays, we have ways to grow airways with oral appliances. I will next review surgical, non-surgical, well-known, and lesser-known therapies that have proven effectiveness for all levels of sleep issues.

Surgical Therapies

Implant: These are medical devices placed under the skin in a surgical situation at your doctor's office or in a hospital setting. These do not allow the body to heal but create a Band-Aid to symptoms. I have seen many patients get devices like these and who ignore the reasons they have a need to breathe easier. Below, I have mentioned several of these devices, but there are others on the market:

The AIRLIFT device involves an outpatient procedure where small implants are placed around the hyoid bone in the throat to help you keep your airway open by stabilizing the hyoid bone.

The Inspire Device comes with its own remote control. It is an implant surgically placed under the tissue in the chest cavity that will stimulate the vagus nerve to help you breathe when your oxygen is dropping.

THN Sleep Therapy is another implant that delivers stimulation to the tongue during sleep to reduce apnea events.

Tonsillectomy/Adenoidectomy: Another surgical fix for breathing easier at night. Considered for people of all ages when their tonsils are chronically inflamed and enlarged blocking the airway. Adenoid tissue is located above and posterior to the tonsils. These are often clipped at the time of a tonsillectomy to resolve inflammation surgically. Consider that this inflammation is not being addressed through cause and effect with this procedure. In other words, the allergen causing the inflammation is not being rooted out of the life of the patient. This is treating symptoms. The tonsils are actually lymph nodes whose purpose is to collect irritants to the body and excrete them. When they are not present, another body part has to do this work. Sometimes when the airway is increased, these tissues have been found to shrink in size on their own.[12]

Uvulectomy: This involves surgery to remove the uvula in order to raise the height of the roof of the palate adjacent to the airway. The tissue in this area is very vascular. It is a very painful procedure to undergo.

Because it does not address a cause and effect relationship, the bigger picture is that aging tissue anywhere continues to collapse over time. Initially, I have seen uvulectomies improve sleep quality, but after five years or so, the benefits have greatly diminished. The pain from this procedure is great. Almost one-third of surveyed patients reportedly would not have the procedure if they had known about the post-op pain beforehand. Twenty-three percent of patients surveyed suffered long-term complications including dry mouth, difficulty swallowing, and a feeling of a lump in the throat.[1]

Non-Surgical Therapies

Non-Surgical Laser Therapy Solutions/ Nightlase Procedure with the Lightwalker Laser for Snoring and Sleep Apnea Improvement:

Laser therapies for sleep apnea and snoring are continuing to evolve. Some therapies are used to perform the surgical procedures described above. Healing is more rapid and post-operative discomfort is minimized with lasers because tissue can be cauterized when a laser is employed as a tool.

Some dentists are using the Lightwalker laser, a dual high performance Er: YAG and Nd:YAG laser, for assisting with snoring and sleep issues. The laser is applied to the soft palate, which induces collagen production in the tissue. This is not considered to be a surgical treatment application of the laser. There is no anesthetic needed or bleeding that results. Tissue is not cut away in this procedure. The laser heats the tissue and causes shrinking of the collagen fibers. The results are that the tissues of the soft palate tighten and lift, opening the airway. Typically the treatment regimen involves three sessions with the laser. Results are reported to be an average improvement of 85% after three sessions, with 51% improvement after a single session.[2]

CPAP Appliance Therapy stands for Continuous Positive Airway Pressure

It's the most recognized appliance for sleep. It has been used in the sleep appliance industry since the late 1970's/early 1980's when Dr. Colin Sullivan began using positive air pressure though the nose to help open blocked airways. By 1990, the self-sealing bubble mask was introduced, and more patients began using the device for better sleep. By 2014, one million people were using CPAP regularly in the USA.[3] CPAP has been the main medical industry go-to appliance for snoring and sleep apnea. In years past, a physician would write the patient a prescription to purchase one. CPAP works by offering a continuous source of air into the airway by pumping a stream though a mask. Some models have the feature of being able to offer variable rates of air being pumped into the body.[4] One of the main problems with CPAP is that it does not open the airway. So, no matter the depth of how much an airway is crimped, CPAP pumps air into it. So CPAP is a Band-Aid to address symptoms of poor response to breathing naturally.

CPAP has a thirty-five percent long-term success because many patients simply cannot wear the device comfortably. Contraindications for CPAP therapy occur in patients who have:[4,5]

- Copious respiratory secretions
- Severe nausea frequently with vomiting
- Air leak syndrome (pneumothorax with broncho-pleural fistula)
- Facial, esophageal, or gastric surgery
- Trauma or burns involving the face
- Unstable cardiorespiratory status or respiratory arrest
- Reduced consciousness and inability to protect their airway
- Anxious patients (those who may be claustrophobic)
- Severe air-trapping diseases with asthma or chronic obstructive pulmonary disease (COPD)

That list above comprises a lot of very sick people who need to breathe.

Oral Appliance Therapy (OAT)

This is where the dentist can help with sleep.

Oral appliances are a great solution for many who suffer from sleep apnea, and these have excellent compliance from patients. Oral sleep appliances have wide range success. There are different options depending on the sleep symptoms from which you are suffering.

Oral appliances have been found to be as effective for mild and moderate sleep apnea as a CPAP.[5] Oral sleep appliance solutions are an example of solution based integrative dental medicine.

There are some facial profiles that are correlated in some populations with sleep apnea. Types of faces that are suggestive of an underlying sleep apnea diagnosis often belong to those who are overweight (BMI over 25), who have a proportionately short upper lip or who are open-mouthed habitually, and who have an ear that is positioned in front of the shoulder when the patient is sitting or standing up straight.[6]

In the photo below, the patient's ear is anterior to the shoulder:

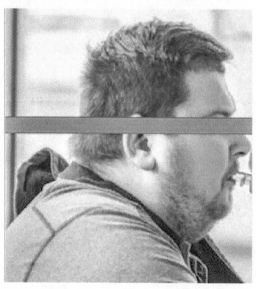

In the illustration above, the patient's ear is positioned in front of (anterior to) the shoulder. Also, there is a double chin and the patient is overweight. His mouth is open, and this may also suggest a habit of mouth breathing rather than nasal breathing.

In the illustration below, the patient's ear is in front of the shoulder, there is a sloped angle from the chin to the chest. This patient has been diagnosed with moderate sleep apnea.

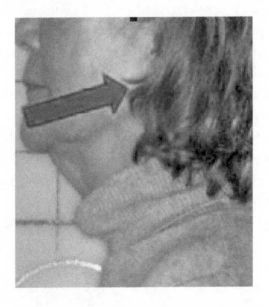

The seam on this patient's sweater correspond to the shoulder. The ear is anterior to the shoulder.

A dentist is wonderfully suited to address the airway because the main constriction is part of the mouth rather than a part of the ears, nose or throat (the part that medicine treats).

Here is an open airway:

The red area depicts the smallest volume of the airway in the patient pictured in a cone beam x-ray below. You may also notice an asymmetry in the way the lower jaw matches up with the upper jaw. The head is

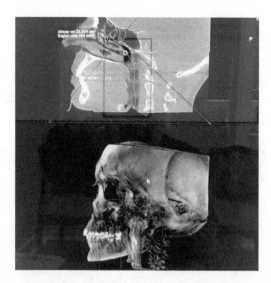

tilted at an angle on the neck. This cone beam is taken when the patient is standing at rest. The smallest part of the airway is the red part, and it is located behind the teeth. This means that the images below depict a patient with severe obstructive sleep apnea. The smallest part of the airway is located behind the teeth, which offers perhaps an easy visual to understand why an oral sleep appliance may be extremely well suited to help minimize the airway size issue. Here is a closed airway:

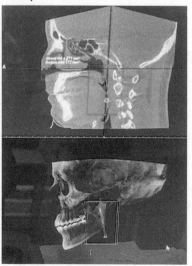

Sometimes the x-ray imaging can show if there can be a reason for neck strain. In the following example, the patient is positioning their head forward and in a lateral position to presumably accommodate for the small airway. The patient pictured in this example has an AHI score over 38, indicating a severe obstructive sleep apnea diagnosis.

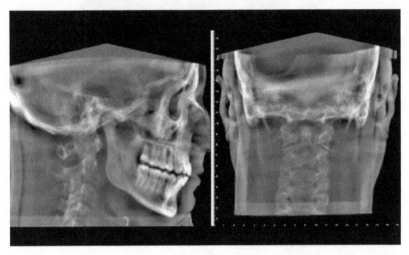

The dental cone beam x-ray can tell us if an oral appliance can help a breathing/sleeping situation by measuring the airway for us and showing us where problems lie.

Oral Appliances Come in Two Classes

1. Those that act as a mandibular repositioner (kind of like a super-effective Band-Aid) and work by holding the patient's lower jaw forward to open the airway.

2. Those that can remodel the airway by functionally shifting the bite of the teeth, altering relationships and crowding between teeth while growing bone using the ligament cells as a platform for this new bone growth. These have been shown to lower AHI, reduce tooth grinding, and improve posture and nasal breathing for kids and adults.[9,10,11,12]

Mandibular Repositioning Appliances Can Act as an Effective Band-Aid Solution to Address Snoring and Sleep Apnea

These are a few of the examples of Type 1 oral appliances (which move the lower jaw forward at night):

A. **The Silent-Nite or Snore Guard (corrects snoring without affecting teeth position or airway):**

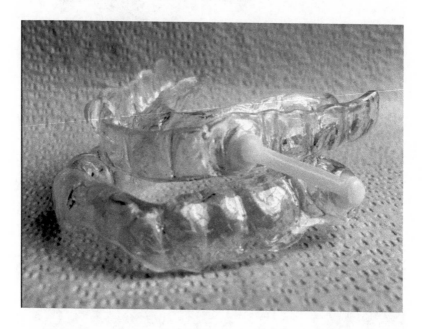

The Silent Nite Appliance works well for mild to moderate sleep issues (not severe sleep apnea) to correct snoring by holding the lower jaw forward.

B. **The TAP (Thornton Adjustable Appliance)** is appropriate for moderate to severe sleep apnea patients who cannot or will not tolerate a CPAP appliance. It will correct snoring as well as maintain an open airway caused by collapsing tissue posterior to the teeth.

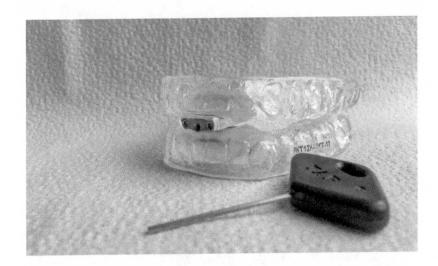

C. **The SUAD**: This device has a lot more hardware than the previous mandibular repositioning appliances shown. It works wonderfully for the individual adult who chooses mandibular advancement therapy and who also has been diagnosed with moderate to severe sleep apnea. These patients may also snore severely.

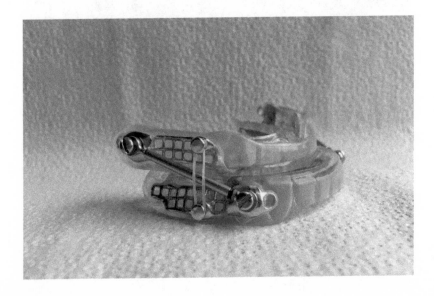

I have found this device to be extremely durable and because of its metal skeleton; they are fairly indestructible if your pet gets ahold of this.

I choose mandibular advancement devices for my patients who have not had and/or who decline to have a sleep test done but have issues with snoring and tooth grinding.

Next, there is second class of dental appliances for sleep. These appliances are my absolute favorite because they address sleep issues but also can address pain, headaches, anxiety, and generally unwind people who have suffered concussions and other symptoms. Unlike braces, these generally do not show, and they are easy to clean.

Also, unlike orthodontic treatment, these functional orthodontic appliances:

- Do not call for tooth extractions to create room for teeth
- Do not put pressure primarily onto teeth but encourage the body's full growth potential
- Can help develop airway girth while addressing bite and crowding issues

Functional orthodontic types of appliances that I use include the ALF, the Oral DNA (by Vivos), and Healthy Start:

D. **ALF therapy (www.ALFtherapy.com)** is an abbreviation for Acute Lightwire Force therapy. Dr. Darick Nordstrom, DDS pioneered the ALF in the late 1970's.

The ALF alleviates upper air resistance, grows the palate in breadth, and alleviates a number of emotional issues such as anxiety because its structure attracts the tongue to the roof of the mouth which promotes parasympathetic nervous system stimulus. These appliances are great for young children to adults.

A photo of an upper ALF appliance:

As the ALF is individualized, there are many treatment designs. For a serious grinder, the appliance may also cover the biting surfaces of teeth.

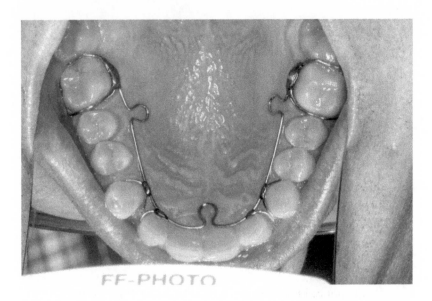

FF-PHOTO

"Its goal is to harness an integration of orthodontic and orthopedic principles to provide health, beauty, and function to the wearer. The ALF creates an aesthetic smile as well as to create for the bones and tissues of the face a functionally comfortable situation. It uses a wire that is nickel-free that attracts the tongue to the roof of the mouth. The wire is applied to the teeth but directs forces to the bone, muscles, and soft tissues of the jaws and face, especially the tongue. For a growing child but also for adults, these forces along the cranial sutures encourage proper bone growth and formation while stabilizing the muscles involved. This results in proper tooth alignment, a good dental bite, and better living. In adults, the light forces along the joints between the bones of the head and neck may result in function for a structurally challenged person."[7]

The ALF appliance helps address restoring function the body does not have. Sometimes this poor function happens when there is a birth trauma, concussion, or a trauma to the breathing apparatus in childhood or from an accident. This disturbed function can cause neural pathways to shut down or to operate in an abnormal way. The patient stops developing or functioning as they once could have. Sometimes, this function is the cause that contributes to sleep dysfunction. Because the appliance helps to establish a new equilibrium in the patient, the patient does not relapse when active treatment is complete and functions healthily post treatment.

Patients who would benefit from ALF might have or have had the following:

- Birth trauma
- Concussion or a fall
- Chronic headaches, shoulder aches, low back pain
- Ringing in the ears, hearing loss
- Sleep disturbances
- Crooked teeth
- Asymmetrical face
- History of relapsed orthodontics
- Possible history of ADD or ADHD
- Possible history of bedwetting
- Any of the above combined with postural issues or habitual slouching

E. **Oral DNA by Vivos** (www.Vivoslife.com)

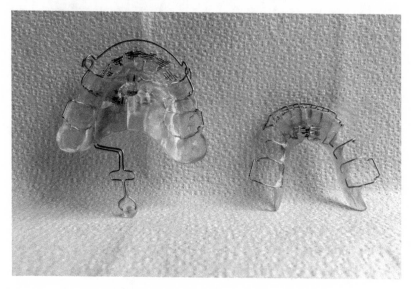

Those who might wear this revolutionary device often overlap with the population who benefits from an ALF device (which means most of the population). The Oral DNA is FDA approved for remodeling the sleep airway to ease sleep and overall opening of the airway, particularly the area of the airway behind or slightly above the teeth (as seen on the cone beam x-rays). These appliances have been tested in children and adults through age seventy years. Vivos Life Corporation has restructured the organization of the dental labs and forces that created Oral DNA and has brought this device to the market today under the Vivos brand name.

The Healthy Start Appliance (www.thehealthystart.com)

This is typically made as a series of several devices for kids to wear. Typical kids who are good candidates for this device are those who have dental crowding, bite issues, airway constrictions, and habits such as thumb sucking or wetting the bed at night. Other kids who may have bedwetting, ADD, ADHD, nervousness, chronic allergies or eczema, headaches, swollen tonsils, or adenoids will often see reduction in these symptoms after wearing these devices for few short weeks during sleep. Some of the devices in this line are habit-correcting. These are worn mostly at night during sleep. They also promote a good night's sleep while harnessing growth potential in the child. These devices are BPA-free, silicone- and latex-free. There is not a photo included here of the devices because there are so many. Some are similar to others pictured earlier in this chapter.

Treatment Considerations to Choose an Oral Device

To screen a patient, I make sure patients have:

A cone beam x-ray so we can see where an obstruction to the airway may lie. Sometimes there is actually a sinus issue that is not a dental problem. In that case, a referral to my ENT colleagues makes sense.

Dental models and many photographs are made to appreciate the anatomical uniqueness of the patient and fully appreciate what design the appliance may have built into it to support the patient in their individualized way.

A polysomnograph (sleep study) is recorded, either through a take-home device or by sending the patient to a sleep center for evaluation. A physician reads and diagnoses the sleep condition. Now, the dentist can get to work if a patient prefers an oral appliance over CPAP or surgery. If a patient has already had a sleep study less than two years prior to their dental visit, we can use the evidence from that study to shape a treatment plan of action.

Other Considerations

An appointment for education. We set aside about ninety minutes to educate patients, collect the date listed above, and to answer questions. We also look at some standard test panels for documenting the patient's perception of the sleep concerns present.

Clues that a dental patient may have a sleep disorder is a dental history of:

- Breaking down teeth to warrant the need for dental crown work, implants, or extractions from cracked teeth

- Mallampati Score over a "1." This score is a reflection of tissue anatomy and inflammation in the back of the throat with can contribute to a compromised airway. Scores range from 1-4.[8]

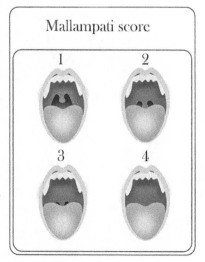

In the photo on below, the patient has a Mallampati score of a 2 or 3.

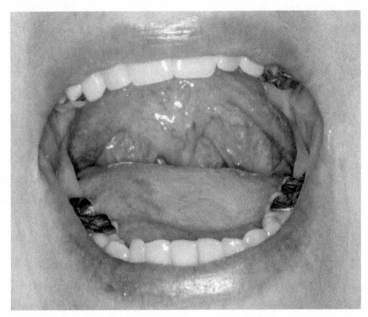

- Extra bone, called a torus or tori, that can be located on either the maxilla (roof of the mouth) or on mandible, usually behind the teeth.
- Second molars (the most posterior teeth) are tipped towards the cheek in relation to the other teeth as in the lower picture shown in this photograph:

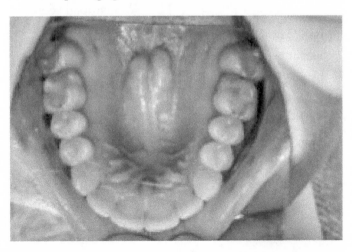

Tongue and Lip Ties

We also evaluate the patient with a very extensive head and neck exam. We look to see if the patient may be tongue- or lip-tied. These ties are a name given to the situation when the frenum, a muscle attachment between the tongue and lower jaw or between the lip and the gum tissue, are abnormally short, which restricts the natural movement of the soft tissue. For babies, it has become increasingly familiar with pediatricians that tongue and lip ties can create difficulty for babies who are nursing. Sometimes, it is helpful for tongue and lip ties to be clipped to restore proper soft tissue function to the mouth and tongue. The patient below is severely tongue tied and cannot stick his tongue outside of his mouth. He has a very small airway, sleep apnea, and reports that his wife hears him when he periodically stops breathing while sleeping throughout the night.

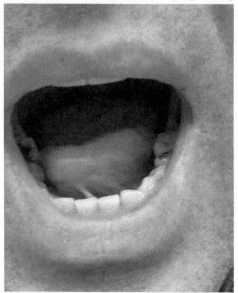

Oral appliances can help with sleep and help treatment issues beyond sleep such as:

Parkinson's Disease, Tourette's Syndrome, and TMJ pain. Oral appliances for these issues often are geared towards opening the bite for patients with constricted airflow. They can often help reduce the symptoms of syndromes that can be in part caused by crimped nerve and airway tissue. One such device is called the GELB appliance, after its inventor. These devices can be likened to orthotics for shoes in people who have issues with their feet or gait.

How to know if your family members may have a sleep issue: For danger signs and symptoms in kids and co-workers, see the list below, labeled for kids (who are just young people).

Symptoms of Kids Who Likely Have Sleep Issues Currently or Will Develop Sleep Issues Over Time (from Sally Fallon, Weston A. Price Foundation)[13]

- Crooked teeth and v-shape instead of u-shape arches
- Dark circles under eyes and/or whites of eyes showing above or below the iris of eye
- Recurrent ear infections
- Birth trauma
- History of a fall, head trauma, broken nose
- Poor eyesight
- Snoring
- Morning dry mouth or very stinky breath
- Daytime tiredness or hyperactivity
- Allergies, eczema, chronic stuffy nose
- Mouth breathing
- ADD/ADHD
- Bedwetting
- Poor posture and general failure to thrive, pot belly
- Asymmetrical face
- Learning problems
- Pituitary gland issues

- Thumb sucking
- Teeth grinding
- Open bite (teeth in front are not overlapping and tongue often fits in that space, usually when patient swallows)
- Deep bite (where the upper front teeth cover the lower front teeth almost completely when the patient bites down)
- Under bite (lower teeth are set back from upper teeth –buck teeth)
- Mismatched midline of the teeth in relation to the face
- Lower teeth that fit in front of the upper teeth (cross bite)
- Small chin or weak chin (chin is not protruded when patient turns sideways)
- Narrow nostrils or where one is larger than the other
- Uneven ears
- Forward head (ears should be over the shoulders when patient is standing erect)
- Jaw that opens up in a crooked fashion
- A very long face or very flat face
- Tourette's syndrome
- Nervous ticks
- Chronically chapped lips
- Not having space between the posterior baby teeth
- Tongue that has imprints of teeth on the sides
- History of chipped or broken teeth
- Extra bone growing in roof or in jaws (maxillary or mandibular torus)
- History of needing a lot of dental work
- In an adult, include PMS or ED (erectile dysfunction)
- Hashimoto's or thyroid issues

A good time for a screening is by the age of seven or eight years. At this time, the jaws are still quite pliable, and growth can easily be encouraged.

Clues for adults that may suffer from a restricted airway are generally the same as for kids.

What your personal result can look like:

After 18 months of wearing an oral appliance in the evening and during sleeping hours, the patient below has a remodeled airway, as evidenced by a shift away from the red and orange colorations in Exhibit A (Before) and Exhibit B (After 18 months of treatment):

Exhibit A:

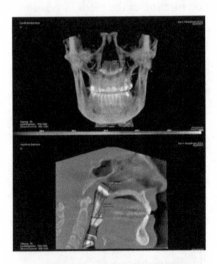

Exhibit B:

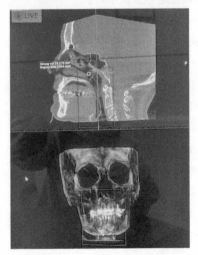

How to Obtain a Diagnosis for Yourself

Seek a dentist in your area who provides services such as ALF, Vivos, Healthy Start. In Atlanta, I am the only dentist who provides all three services for patients of all ages. I prefer offering each device because these truly need to be customized to fit the personality and lifestyle of the patient. When working with an office only offering one type of care, it would be likely that the patient is crammed into a treatment module that may not be best suited for them. Cost ranges from $1,800 to $8,500, depending on severity and number of phases of treatment. One piece of good news is that medical insurance (but not Medicare or Medicaid) will often cover a significant portion of either ALF or Oral DNA therapy.

Using Oral Appliances for Treating Snoring, Sleep and Airway

In summary, oral appliances can address the cause behind sleep issues. Some can hold a patient to their current state so teeth and airway do not worsen in their condition. Others can improve the situation so the patient reaches a new state of equilibrium permanently. I love these functional appliances that promote overall best health conditions for patients. On average, treatment time and cost for functional appliances is about the same cost as traditional orthodontics, and this is covered often by both medical and dental insurance.

Chapter 10:

Integrative Approaches to Uncover Your Best Sleep

"I can think. I can sleep. I can move.
I can ride my bike. I can dream."
— Bill Walton

When you are informed about all sleep solution possibilities, you have your best chance of successful nighttime rest.

Because sleep is diagnosed by physicians but can be treated by dentists and because a lot of times there is a history of trauma or nutritional deficiencies, getting you the best results for the best sleep is often a team effort.

Integrative healthcare is where there is a collaborative effort to get patients the solutions they need. It approaches each patient as an individual. In my dental office, we work closely with integrative physicians, osteopaths, chiropractors, psychologists, nutritionists, and a local farmers market to deliver an individualized approach to health and sleep.

When the body is functioning optimally, sleep, nutrition, and health are present. Decay in teeth is a rarity. Periodontal disease ceases to be present. Inflammation in the body is minimized, and good sleep is a regular occurrence. Trauma, either physical or emotional, is addressed.

What we also know is that teeth, in other branches of medicine such as traditional Chinese Medicine, are connected to meridians, or energy pathways. When there is dental pain or trauma, often there is a connection emotionally or to another organ. Integrative dentistry connects these concepts and events for patients so that they can begin to sort through the causative nature of their disease. When you address the cause, you are more likely to work out a more equitable solution for the long-term and live a healthier life.

Below is a diagram adapted from a variety of sources on the relationship between the meridians and teeth:[1]

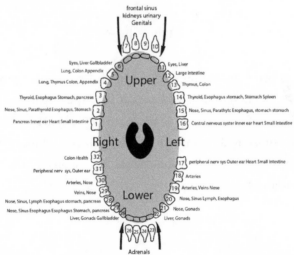

Some research has even suggested that there are relationships between the teeth and emotions. One study observed that up to thirty-seven percent of people observed showed symptoms of a negative mood alteration that correlated directly with oral health status. In particular, the participants who scored the worst in emotional state had the worst oral health status. In particular, their mood was one of more aggression and fatigue. In another survey, over half of adults with teeth reported that they had been affected emotionally in some way by their teeth. In eight percent of those cases, the impact was considered by the patient to have significantly reduced their quality of life.[1,2]

We need more empirical studies to better understand this relationship between teeth and emotions. On a personal note, I can attest that often a dental tooth ache seems to occur in a patient's life when they are already stressed out, which is especially interesting to me because the physical cause of the tooth ache (decay or developing abscess) will often have been present for many months before the onset of actual pain.

Some research has even suggested that there are relationships between the teeth and emotions.

Meridian	Teeth	Emotions
Heart	1,16,17, 32 (wisdom teeth)	Loneliness, Acute Grief, Humiliation, Feeling Trapped, Inhibition, Lack of Joy, Greed, Feeling Unlovable
Small Intestines	1,16,17, 32 (wisdom teeth)	Loneliness, Acute Grief, Humiliation, Feeling Trapped, Inhibition, Lack of Joy, Greed, Feeling Unlovable
Circulation /Sex	1,16,17, 32 (wisdom teeth)	Loneliness, Acute Grief, Humiliation, Feeling Trapped, Inhibition, Lack of Joy, Greed, Feeling Unlovable

Triple Warmer/ Endocrine	1, 16, 17, 32 (wisdom teeth)	Loneliness, Acute Grief, Humiliation, Feeling Trapped, Inhibition, Lack of Joy, Greed, Feeling Unlovable
Spleen/ Pancreas	2,3,14,15,21,20, 28, 29 (upper molars and lower premolars)	Anxiety, Self-Punishment, Broken Power, Low Self Worth, Obsession
Stomach	2,3,14,15,21,20, 28, 29 (upper molars and lower premolars)	Anxiety, Self-Punishment, Broken Power, Low Self Worth, Obsession
Lung	4,5,12,13,18,19,30,31 (upper premolars and lower molars)	Chronic Grief, Overcritical, Sadness, Controlling, Feeling Trapped, Dogmatic, Compulsive, Uptight
Large Intestine	4,5,12,13,18,19,30,31 (upper premolars and lower molars)	Chronic Grief, Overcritical, Sadness, Controlling, Feeling Trapped, Dogmatic, Compulsive, Uptight
Liver	6,11,22,27 (canine teeth)	Anger, Resentment, Frustration, Blaming, Cannot Take Action, Manipulation
Gallbladder	6,11,22,27 (canine teeth)	Anger, Resentment, Frustration, Blaming, Cannot Take Action, Manipulation
Kidney	7,8,9,10,23,24,25,26 (upper and lower incisors)	Fear, Shame, Guilt, Broken Will, Shyness, Helplessness, Deep Exhaustion
Bladder	7,8,9,10,23,24,25,26 (upper and lower incisors)	Fear, Shame, Guilt, Broken Will, Shyness, Helplessness, Deep Exhaustion

Source: Chart info from Ralph Wilson (www.NaturalWorldHealing.com), based upon the work of Deitrich Klinghardt, MD (www.Klinghardt.org and www.NeuralTherapy.com) Louisa Williams, www.RadicalMedicine.com.

The Oral, Whole-Body, and Sleep Repercussions of History of a Head Injury and/or Birth Trauma

Remember my personal story about my daughter who fell on a flight of stairs as a young girl? It was after her fall that her dad and I noticed that she had started snoring horribly. It turns out that the fall not only caused my daughter to need stitches in her chin but also that she had suffered cranial nerve trauma, which was connected to the onset of her snoring and poor sleep. The snoring caused us to revisit her pediatrician with many questions for months after the stitches in her chin had healed. Why was she snoring? The initial suggestion was: "Well you turned on your furnace" or that "there could be allergens from seasonal pollen in the air." I noticed that she started needing daytime naps again. She had perpetual dark circles under her eyes. I was getting increasingly frequent calls from her teacher at school that she could not focus and complete classwork.

Then the suggestion was, "Perhaps she broke her nose, but we don't address this until she is a teenager." A homemade video tape of her loud snoring and my pressing led me to a visit with an ENT for children. The diagnosis was that my daughter's tonsils and adenoids were enlarged and that she would benefit from their removal. In 2006, this seemed to be the best choice. With today's dental offerings, I would choose differently for my daughter. Nowadays, I recommend that patients in this situation seek out an oral appliance and a teamwork approach from some of the following health practitioners: an osteopath for cranial-sacral work, a chiropractor, and possibly a myo-functional therapist to help reset the cranial nerves and tongue habits. When you unwind a patient from trauma, sleep, mental acuity, and focus can all improve.

Cranial nerves that have suffered trauma may chronically affect stress experienced by the human body. There are twelve pairs of cranial nerves. These are formed differently from all the other nerves in the spinal cord. We refer to the twelve pairs of cranial nerves in Roman numerals to delineate them from one another. Below is a chart summarizing the twelve cranial nerves, their functions, and notes about how they originate.[4]

Cranial Nerve #	Organ it controls	Origin of nerve	Primitive brain function purpose
I-Olfactory	smell	Extension of brain stem	Examine food
II-Optic	sight	" " " "	Examine food
III-Oculomotor	Moves eyelid, eyeball, pupils, lens	***	***
IV-Trochlear	eyeball	***	***
V-Trigeminal	Facial muscles, teeth, muscles that chew, pain, senses touch to the face	***	***
VI-Abducens	Eyeballs (moves outwards)	***	***
VII-Facial	Taste, tears, saliva, enables movement of facial expressions (ex. The smile)	***	***

VIII-Vestibulo-cochlear	Hearing and Balance (Auditory), also smooth heart muscles (esp. atrial function)	***	
IX. Glossopha-ryngeal	Swallowing, sali-vary flow, taste	***	
X-Vagus	Control of Parasympathetic N.S., muscles in GI tract, heart-beat, breathing, tongue	***	
XI-Accessory	Moving head and shoulders, swallowing	***	
XII-Hypoglossal	Tongue mus-cles, speech, swallowing	***	

*** Cranial nerves III-VII all have origins in both the primitive brain stem as well as in the cerebral cortex which developed later evolutionarily.

As the primitive brain developed in evolution-expanding and developing additional regions, it is thought that the cerebral cortex formed with the function of analyzing material outside of the brain and drawing conclusions about this material. The cerebrum of the brain constituted the ability for higher thought and discernment. Thus, cranial nerves III, IV, V, VI, and VII have parts deriving from the brain stem and the cerebrum. These two parts are wrapped together and go forth to the organ and tissue innervated. Therefore, nerves III, IV, V, VI, and VII have both sensory and motor abilities wrapped together. (They are woven from indirectly from the brain stem for sensory ability *with* motor ability that goes to the opposite side of the brain, whereas the nerves I and II only sensory fibers from the brain stem.) Also, it is notable that these two parts of the nerves in III through VII have a part of sensing on the same side of the body that they are located on (the sensory part) and a motor part that controls the opposite side of the body from where it originates from the brain (the motor part).

It is thought that the original primitive brain regulated intake and out-take of the body and that there was one opening for both eating (intake) and elimination of waste products (outtake). For this reason, the motor nerve fibers going to the opposite side of the body are paired with the cranial nerve that contains sensory fibers on same side the cranial nerve is located. In the primitive brain, the left side of the body controlled elimination and the right side of the brain controlled food and respiratory (breathing) intake.

When you consider a head injury or a traumatic birthing process in a person's medical history, it becomes more understandable why what was a little head trauma potentially many years ago may have dramatic impact on one's development and sense of self and ability in the world. Make sure that you always disclose to your health provider that you have a history of a head or birth trauma, even if you are not sure of the significance of this information.

You see, just because a head trauma took place many years ago does not mean healing has ever completely occurred. This may be visible, for example, in a patient who suffers a stroke after a head injury or a baby who has had learning disabilities attributed to a difficult labor of the mother. But sometimes, skeletal strains associated with blunt trauma can occur and just never unwind.

As Sir Isaac Newton discovered and determined as the Third Law of Motion, "for every action, there is a reaction!" Imagine you hit a piñata with a bat. The piñata swings in the air and perhaps the stick succeeds with a penetrating blow to the interior filled with candy, which proceeds to fall onto the ground. Now, let's say someone hits you with the same bat! You feel the impact on one side of your head, and your neck potentially takes your head back. Your torso may reel away from the unexpected impact of the blow. You feel immediate pain and dizziness, and maybe a bruise or swollen place is visible a minute or so after the incident. Later, maybe you see a little protrusion on your forehead you didn't remember before the incident. But you may not appreciate that there could be a place that is still healing under the skin and bone, down to the nerve.

I always recommend the patient visits a healthcare practitioner after a head injury. Also, if you have suffered head trauma, please have a doctor or dentist perform a cranial nerve exam on you so that you can know if there are any nerves that have become lazy or are not fully functioning after an injury. Frequently, after such an exam, the test activity for the nerve can also be a healing way to bring the nerve back into alignment. For example, someone with a constricted airway from a near-drowning incident may unknowingly be unable to have a light touch to the uvula. A light touch to the uvula in such a person could produce an episode of instant trauma, including tears or even pain somewhere else in the body. In such a person, using a long Q-tip to touch the uvula can help to settle the fear of drowning again. It may sincerely ease everyday breathing while the vagus nerve learns to settle down and not be on vigilant mode.

And this brings us to the sympathetic and parasympathetic nervous nystems. The sympathetic nervous system is often referred to as one's fight or flight response, such as one would have needed in prehistoric times if one needs to run from a tiger in the jungle. The parasympathetic nervous system is the nervous system that kicks on after you have successfully gotten away from the tiger. Now, you can recharge with rest and by eating so that you will be strong for when the next time the tiger finds you.

In most parts of today's world, there are not tigers chasing individuals in the jungle. What we do have, however, is the self-induced stress notifications from our alarm clocks, deadlines, lack of sleep, and social troubles. We do not take proper time to recharge and to rest. We eat often on the go, and many times the food is of inflammatory and soft texture nature. The inflammation from stress and poor diet creates depletion of vitamin stores in the body, which then does not allow us a proper parasympathetic recharge. The bite of many modern-day kids is not well formed due to softer diets. The narrow dental arch and palate drives the tongue into a downward posture. Medical research shows that this downward tongue posture actually adversely affects the heart.

With relation to the mouth, the tongue is the second muscle to develop after the heart in utero. The vagus nerve (cranial nerve X) regulates the heartbeat. Medical research shows that when the tongue is positioned in a downward place (not up against the palate behind the teeth with the lips closed at rest), the sympathetic nervous system is put into overdrive constantly. This decreases HRV (heart rate variability), making the heart work harder than it should.[3]

Also, what I have witnessed in a lot of head injury cases is that cranial nerve VII can get shut down from normal functioning because the injury causes overdrive of the sympathetic nervous system. When a provider can help the patient reawaken cranial nerve VII's normal function, the sympathetic nervous system gets calmed and more normal cranial nerve function can be restored.

Case Study: The Conclusion of Sarah's Story

Sarah is my daughter who snored. After her tonsils and adenoids were removed, some changes happened. Sarah did have a growth spurt after the tonsils were removed, but she had focus issues (ADD-like symptoms) at school. We did not wish for our daughter to be labeled with a diagnosis about her learning issues. We sought nutrition and healing through playing outside with a new puppy and being physically active. Sarah also took to playing the violin and could actually memorize concertos by first grade. We did massages at night before bedtime and vitamin supplements with a drink to idealize Sarah's levels of nutrition for best healing from her fall. You can see in the photo below that Sarah had some of the classic signs of potential sleep apnea: an underdeveloped upper jaw, dark circles under her eyes, the whites showing under the irises of her eyes, and a small lower jaw. She developed very crowded teeth by the second grade, and orthodontics were placed to straighten Sarah's teeth. The orthodontic appliance helped to expand Sarah's jaw, and this correlated with our daughter beginning to have an easier time in school academically. The snoring became a seldom occurrence. The allergies mostly have resolved too. Sarah became more at ease as she got better sleep and good nutrition. At the age of fifteen, new functional orthodontic appliances (combination of Vivos' Oral DNA and ALF) were used to continue to promote jaw growth and remodeling of the airway.

Below is a photo of Sarah at age five and another at age seventeen. From the material discussed earlier in this book, you may now be able to identify some aspects of Sarah's visual appearance that indicates she may have sleep issues at the age of five.

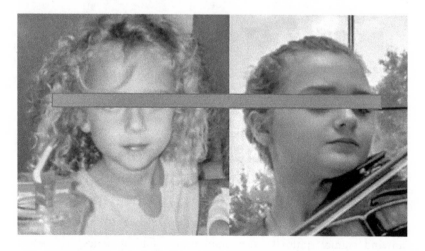

The sympathetic and parasympathetic nervous systems are shown in the following diagrams. When we sense stress, our body up-regulates our sympathetic nervous system.

Repeated and prolonged stress shortens our telomeres and shortens our lifespan because blood flow to certain organs is increased and chemicals in the HPA axis are released to help us cope with the stress. Being able to up-regulate the parasympathetic nervous system is helpful to enable us to age our best. We sleep better when our parasympathetic nervous system is often engaged.

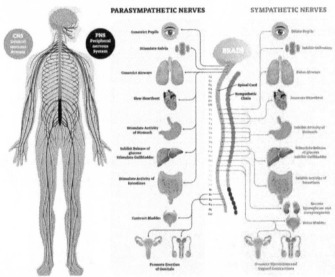

Having self-awareness to recharge with food, drink and rest can reset us for our parasympathetic nervous system to become our more prevailing way of living.

A Note About Osteopathic Work, Cranial Sacral Osteopathy, Chiropractics, and Massage Post Traumatic Brain Injury

Osteopathy (and cranial osteopathy) is a science that looks to gently unwind cranial traumas from brain injury. Chiropractics or massage therapy may also achieve similar results. Cranial osteopathy, particularly, looks and feels like getting a massage, but it helps to move interstitial fluid throughout the body and unblock or ease the flow of stagnant tissue. Frequently, a result of such therapy can help unwind an upper spine or postural strain. Such strains can affect the levelness of shoulders, hips, arches of feet, and the bite (occlusion) of the teeth. Generally, this technique facilitates an extremely gentle healing process for all age groups after either birth trauma or head injury.

In my area just outside of Atlanta, I have found an enthusiastic pediatrician, Dr. Arlene Dijamco, M.D., who uses cranial sacral osteopathic therapy as a tool to reset the parasympathetic nervous system in patients who have had physical trauma. The results have been truly amazing. Dr. Dijamco is pictured below working on a patient. She spends time outside of her office volunteering at trauma sites (such as post-earthquake sites) to help people move forward after a stressful event.

Cranial sacral therapy originated in the United States and was pioneered by William Sutherland almost one hundred years ago. Research supports that can be extremely effective in decreasing pain, improving mental cognition and memory, increasing sleeptime, and improving sleep quality after concussions in professional football players from the NFL and Canadian Football League who had been medically diagnosed with post-concussion syndrome after ten treatment sessions over a three-month period.[14]

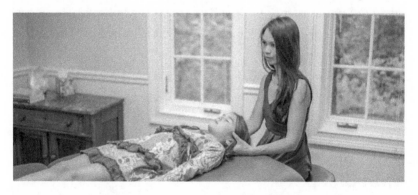

Dr. Arlene Dijamco, M.D. exhibiting cranial osteopathy

You can use exercise, sleep, and meditation for ultimately healing yourself from the past and upregulate your parasympathetic nervous system! And the exercise mentioned here can be achieved in many forms. Exercise resets how our bodies process the energy and nutrients from food and helps us heal and age better. For some, yoga has been found to be as effective as physical therapy for healing from chronic pain.[6]

Generally speaking, adapting a variety of exercises in your regimen will keep you more interested and will help you kick over into parasympathetic nervous system (either during the restful parts of a yoga routine – shavasana – or post cardio workout).

Sleep

Establishing a proper sleep routine can go a ways towards getting proper rest. This can include establishing a regular bed time, using essential oils such as lavender on your pillowcase, or soaking in a bath of Epsom salts (magnesium sulfate).

Anxiety is a common ailment preventing quality sleep for many of us, and it can interfere with getting the rest your body requires to function at its best. Screen time and bright blue lights (as contained in fluorescent bulbs and computer and TV screens) have been shown to interfere with our internal clocks and circadian rhythms. Wearing orange (blue light blocking) glasses later in the evening reportedly helps some people ease into restful sleep better. Room-darkening curtains in the bedroom can also help promote sleep.

For those who suffer from post-traumatic stress disorder, your REM (deep sleep or rapid eye movement sleep) sleep can be affected by your PTSD as well as your memory.[8]

Role of Oral Myofunctional Therapy (OMT) with Sleep

Oral myofunctional therapy is not speech therapy. Speech therapy is a part of oral myofunctional therapy. Oral myofunctional therapy will strengthen muscle segments of the tongue and oral structures so they function optimally and support the swallow, breathing and bone formation and support of the face. I suggest for patients who have issues from suffering many troubles, some of which include:

Oral Sleep Apnea and Snoring

- Post stroke
- Post-concussion therapy
- Birth trauma
- Reverse swallow or tongue and/or lip tie history
- Children who are super picky eaters (often indicates a tongue or lip tie)

OMT can teach people of all ages how to use their tongue and facial muscles in their best way. There are eight segments to the tongue and many muscles that enable one to smile. OMT is an effective adjunct treatment when used with an oral appliance to reduce the severity of sleep apnea and snoring because it helps to reshape the muscles surrounding the airway. When used in adults, it has been proven to reduce the AHI, RDI, reduce daytime sleepiness, and improve sleep quality. In children with residual apnea, OMT has been found to promote a decrease of AHI, increase oxygen saturation, and improve muscle tone of tissue surrounding the airway.[9]

A tongue thrust is a habit that affects the way someone swallows and frequently is a symptom of the tongue being in a downward position. Heart rate variability is reduced by a tongue thrust.

The most common reason I refer patients for OMT is because of a tongue thrust that I can see will negatively impact oral appliance therapy. When I refer a patient to a myofunctional therapist, I can expect to correct or at least minimize a tongue thrust, and the patient learns to use more equally/symmetrically the muscles that enable speech and swallowing. When it comes to unwinding trauma or straightening teeth, myofunctional therapy can help a patient speed through therapy and not relapse after functional oral appliance treatment such as with ALF, Vivos, or Healthy Start appliances.

Here are one patient's before and (three months) after starting a myofunctional therapy program:

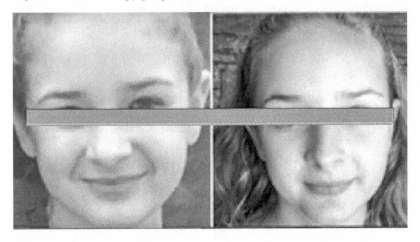

Three months after beginning myofunctional therapy, the patient above has experienced significant facial growth. The therapy supports growth of the maxilla (upper jawbone) and encourages placement of the tongue against the roof of the mouth, which results in a filling out of the cheekbones. The tissue folds (nasolabial folds) between the cheeks and the lips are less pronounced after three months of therapy. A course of therapy often lasts about six months. This patient had habitually breathed through her mouth before OMT and had adapted nose breathing while sleeping by the end of her therapy.

Myofunctional therapy improves sleep quality and duration. In a study of two groups of children who had been previously diagnosed with sleep apnea, group one experienced myofunctional therapy after tonsillectomy and adenoidectomy versus and the other group of children who had undergone tonsillectomy and adenoidectomy and did not experience post-operative myofunctional therapy. The result of the study was that the group of kids with myofunctional therapy did not relapse into sleep apnea.

In another study comparing myofunctional therapy versus oral splinting at night, myofunctional therapy led to a reduction of muscle pain. Also, myofunctional therapy has been found to improve jaw muscle strength and range of motion. Clinically, when patients struggle at dental appointments and with cleaning their own teeth, there is often a component of limited mouth-opening ability. Patients I have seen who have undergone myofunctional therapy are able to clean their teeth with more ease. Children are less picky eaters after myofunctional therapy.[6,7]

How does oral myofunctional therapy differ from speech therapy? OMT addresses many health issues including speech issues. It is a fuller program than speech therapy.

Myo Munchee

One more note about oral myofunctional therapy… I often incorporate the use of an over-the-counter device called the Myo Munchee, from Australia with my patient undergoing OMT. The creator of the Myo Munchee, Dr. Kevin Bourke, was a dentist. The device was originally used as an adjunct to help kids improve oral hygiene. The device was to be worn, generally speaking, for several short rounds of treatment daily. The device has small nubby "bristles" to scrub teeth. Oral pH of the mouth rises with this activity, and saliva glands are stimulated. The device also works the muscles of the mouth when used as a chewing tool. The MyoMunchee company does have some promising research supporting using the device in conjuction with OMT to help teeth straighten to some degree and for decreasing AHI (improving sleep testing results).[15]

Using Exercise, Sleep, and Meditation for Healing Is Upregulating Your Parasympathetic Nervous System

Exercise

Resets how our bodies use food and helps us heal, age better. Yoga in a classroom has been found for some to be as effective as physical therapy for healing from chronic pain.

Generally speaking, adapting a variety of exercises in your regimen will keep you more interested; it will help you kick over into parasympathetic nervous system (either during the restful parts of a yoga routine– shavasana – or post-cardio work out).[8]

Sleep

Establishing a proper sleep routine can go a long way toward getting proper rest. This can include establishing a regular bedtime, using essential oils such as lavender on your pillowcase, or soaking in a bath of Epsom salts (magnesium sulfate).

Anxiety is a common ailment preventing quality sleep for many of us, and it can interfere with getting the rest your body requires to function at its best. Screen time and bright blue lights (as contained in fluorescent bulbs and computer and TV screens) have been shown to interfere with our internal clocks and circadian rhythms. Wearing orange (blue light blocking) glasses later in the evening reportedly helps some people ease into restful sleep better. Room-darkening curtains in the bedroom can also help promote sleep.

For those who suffer from post-traumatic stress disorder, your REM (deep sleep or rapid eye movement sleep) sleep can be affected by the PTSD as well as memory.[10]

Other Medical Devices That Might Bring a Patient Comfort

Chi machines or lymphatic drainage systems

These are machines available over the internet under various names that use vibration to drain lymphatics. The research around the lymphatic system is gaining more attention in the medical community these days. The lymphatic system is extremely important to assisting, healing, and detoxifying processes.[11] This is helpful in those who have suffered a concussion.[12] While more studies need to be done to fully understand the impact of seeking lymphatic drainage from various therapies, these studies are starting to be conducted. So far, we do know that mild lymphatic drainage has been concluded to not be a factor in increasing the risk of breast cancer in patients with breast-cancer-related lymphedema.[13] Patients use this device by lying down on the floor with their ankles in the device. These types of devices retail for around $150.

Rezzi-Max

This device sold on the internet has helped many who have headaches and TMJ pain. The patient uses this at home to massage the head using gentle vibration. Vibratory waves help with mild lymphatic drainage. This is a handheld device, and it retails for around $300.

Case Study: Chronic Pain and Inflammation Patient: Paul the Concussion Patient

Paul had suffered for years from old football injuries from high school and college. His BMI is 30 (one is considered obese in this BMI range). He has had a couple of concussions and works hard to support his family at the age of fifty-one. He doesn't find time to get out and exercise as regularly as he once did. The pain in his neck and shoulders really sets him back in his activity level. His neck size is a seventeen (large neck circumference). He is snoring regularly and occasionally seems to be gasping for air, according to his wife. Sometimes his wife reportedly sleeps in a separate bedroom "just to get better sleep." Paul has tried the benchmark of best sleep therapy, the CPAP, after a sleep study revealed that he does not get good REM sleep and wakes up 11 times hours. Paul wore the CPAP for a few weeks before ditching it due to the discomfort and constriction he felt. He also does some weekend camping and travels and does not want to lug the CPAP around in his carryon and hiking luggage.

Steps and Suggestions for Treatment

1. Sleep test to confirm sleep apnea with a medical doctor: Paul would have more energy to lose weight and would probably feel less chronic pain if we could get him sleeping better. Since his sleep test is over two years old, we had him do a take home sleep test and had this read by his ENT. (A dentist does not diagnose sleep apnea and must engage the consultation of a medical doctor to render the diagnosis of sleep apnea.) Since Paul does have sleep apnea but does not wish to wear a CPAP machine while sleeping, we took a cone beam (also called CBCT scan) of Paul's airway (from the bottom of the orbital rim to the hyoid bone). The scan reveals some degenerative troubles with his TMJ (temporal-mandibular joint) and a military neck (a neck that appears extremely straight on an x-ray, possibly from an old football injury in this case). Since the airway is constricted behind the teeth, we elected to pursue an oral appliance that can be worn while sleeping and for several hours in the evening to help reposition the teeth to decompress the TMJ and that will also expand the airway space. Expanding the airway space should help Paul sleep better.

2. A cranial nerve exam at our dental office revealed a few nerves that seem to respond with a sort of laziness or abnormal slow

response and another that causes a gag response (touching the uvula with a cotton swab). This suggested that Paul may also still have some repercussions from an old concussion injury.

3. We referred Paul to a nearby medical doctor who can perform cranial sacral release and help "unwind" Paul from torsion still present from an old injury. After having seen this doctor several times, Paul said he really is feeling less chronic pain in his neck. He also enrolled in some yoga classes biweekly, which he reported is keeping him more social and increasing his flexibility.

4. We delivered a Vivos appliance to Paul to support his airway while he sleeps at night.

5. Paul was sleeping better within a week of appliance delivery. His dental work is holding up because it is protected while he sleeps. His airway is increasing in size from his Vivos appliance. He is feeling more rested.

6. Paul graduated from active treatment twenty months after we begin. His cone beam reflects a normal airway size. He is able to stand more erect and generally feels younger.

Chapter 11

Imagine the Results When Your Health Wishes Are Honored

*"I'm going to sleep well tonight knowing
that I made the right decision."*
– George Ryan

I n October 2018, I found myself lecturing at the American Dental Association's National Conference in Hawaii. When preparing for the lecture, I was looking for a way to introduce the topic of holistic dentistry (which they had selected for my topic) that would not turn off listeners in the first five minutes of the morning discussion. You see, in dental school we are taught one way to do our profession. Medical schools are teaching one way for health. Anything outside of that will lead the dentist or a variety of other health professions to a place of discredit and falsehood.

Then, I came upon the concept of Ho'oponopono. Ho'oponopono is said to be a reminder to make sincere efforts to understand another person, culture, or country. Historically, since Hawaiians lived on islands, there were not many other places to go for an outcast or someone who disagrees with the bigger community. So, the group of dwellers would commune in Ho'oponopono and determine how a dispute would be resolved. A conclusion would be reached by a group of elders, and the community would convene for a meal after the decision.

If you apply Ho'oponopono to dentistry or other healthcare and you are the healthcare provider, you could find yourself learning to listen more to how a patient wants to pursue treatment when they are sick. As a patient, you might learn to appreciate how each branch of medicine will view your body and suggest treatment. Sometimes, there are resulting holes in treatment as one branch may disregard another health issue as it is not part their scope of care. As a society, we have been treating symptoms within various areas of medical expertise. The treatment choices of the patient will be best served when overall approaches to health are coordinated amongst providers and individualized and unique plans of action are executed on the patient's behalf. I wish that healthcare practitioners would seek more opportunities to learn about new care approaches. When we seek the freedom of choice and have a respect for what a patient desires in their healing journey, the patient can more fully engage in getting well. The healing would cease to be a profit center for corporations and become a process of caring on a personal level, where a relationship between the provider and patient can thrive. The patient would still expect the healthcare provider to educate them on the technique they feel is best. If the patient does not agree with the approach the healthcare provider wishes to use, it would behoove the patient to seek a provider that is a better fit for their desired plan of action.

In applying Ho'oponopono to dentistry, I hope my profession, other professions, and the general public will learn to approach healthcare choices with a more open mind. What is the best course of action for one person is not necessarily the right choice for another. The public needs more access to health options that can fit the varied lifestyles and budgets. Patients are increasingly combining the worlds of healthcare, mixing these up for an individualized approach for wellness and healing. I hope that my colleagues will rise to the new demands of integrative care from their patients. Being able to adapt integrative approaches to care will save costs and can re-humanize the caring feel that should be a part of medical treatment.

The information presented in this book has the potential to help you from day one. Sharing the data in this book can help many who sleep poorly and who need affordable answers for better sleep.

My most hopeful takeaways for you:

- Modern dentistry can offer a widespread integrative approach to uncover the most appropriate solution for addressing sleep needs and to enable the patient to reach their best health.
- Let's grow the integrative dental movement and transform health of the masses by sharing the Core of the Snore Protocol!

Core of the Snore Protocol Recap

1. Try herbs and additional vitamins and dietary changes to naturally aid sleep and cut inflammation.
2. Try over-the-counter methods to establish a bedtime routine.
3. Take a sleep test and get a diagnosis from a physician.
4. Obtain genetics testing for understanding your genetic constitution and evoke changes to support your genes.

5. Collaborate with an integrative dentist to find your best solutions for non-surgical treatment that address the causes of why you do not sleep anatomically or put a stop to worsening of symptoms of poor sleep.

6. Potentially seek care from other health providers in your community to sort through ACE, nutrition, and dietary concerns or other health issues to uncover how you got into poor sleep.

7. Give yourself care and time to heal so you sleep and therefore live better.

Additional Tips

- Learn to vet your provider for education and openness for how you wish to be treated. You deserve NO LESS.

- A stitch in time saves nine: Investing on the front end (addressing causes that lead to worse health conditions) can generally save you from a fate of chronic illness.

- Remember: Try less expensive solutions (like a six-dollar solution) before the expensive ones! You may get improvement, and you will have more information to share with your providers about what your symptoms are by having investigated what is or isn't working for you. This will help any professional meet your needs more efficiently.

I have treated many patients for sleep issues for over twenty years. My repertoire of sleep aid methods has increased and matured through years of experience with thousands of friends and patients and on a personal level with spouse, kids, extended family, and myself. For patients like Susan, introduced at the beginning of this book, the integrative dentist in me can't wait to share solutions to manifest wellness in life.

*All articles and information in this book are for educational purposes only. They are to not to be regarded or relied upon as medical advice. These statements have not been evaluated by the Food and Drug

Administration. This book is not intended to diagnose, cure, treat or prevent any disease. Results may vary per person. Consult your health practitioner if you have health problems.

Acknowledgements

T hank you to my patients, for allowing me to serve you. Thank you also to my dental team, who has supported many new endeavors at the office in the last few years as we implemented many changes at the office so we could be the first office in the Atlanta area to offer, under one roof, all of the oral appliances reviewed in this book. We also offer nutrition advice, gene SNP salivary testing, and make recommendations for lifestyle support to help patients obtain better sleep and whole-body wellness. We have had the pleasure to serve so many wonderful clients of all ages. Thank you to my family and to close friends including Trish, Theresa, Kim, Teresa, Arlene, and Suzanne for hanging, supporting, and scheming with me for a number of years so I could return to work to try new technologies.

Thank you to Angela Lauria and The Author Incubator's team, as well as to David Hancock and the Morgan James Publishing team for helping me bring this book to print.

References

Chapter 2:

1. Doering U. Electro Smog – A Danger To Health. 2007. http://www.drdoering.co.nz/index.php? pr=VoltageShock. Accessed June 30, 2012.
2.. Consumer Reports. "Why Americans Can't Sleep." *Product Reviews and Ratings -Consumer Reports*, www.consumerreports.org/sleep/why-americans-cant-sleep/.
3. "Snoring -Overview and Facts." *Sleep Education*, sleepeducation.org/essentials-in-sleep/snoring/overview-and-facts.
4. SoClean, and About SoClean. "10 Sleep Apnea Facts and Statistics You Should Know." *SoClean*, 13 Dec. 2017, www.soclean.com/sleep-talk/2017/09/07/10-sleep-apnea-facts/.

Chapter 3:

1. Sim JJ, Rasgon SA, Derose SF. Review article: Managing sleep apnoea in kidney diseases. Nephrology (Carlton) 2010;15:146–152.[PubMed]

2. Beecroft JM, Zaltzman J, Prasad R, Meliton G, Hanly PJ. Impact of kidney transplantation on sleep apnoea in patients with end-stage renal disease. Nephrol Dial Transplant. 2007;22:3028–3033. [PubMed]

3. Kutner NG. Quality of life and daily hemodialysis. Semin Dial. 2004;17:92–98. [PubMed]

4. Argekar P, Griffin V, Litaker D, Rahman M. Sleep apnea in hemodialysis patients: risk factors and effect on survival. Hemodial Int. 2007;11:435–441. [PubMed]

5. Novak M, Shapiro CM, Mendelssohn D, Mucsi I. Diagnosis and management of insomnia in dialysis patients. Semin Dial. 2006;19:25–31. [PubMed]

6. Unruh ML. Sleep apnea and dialysis therapies: things that go bump in the night? Hemodial Int. 2007;11:369–378. [PubMed]

7. "Sleep Bruxism Related to Obstructive Sleep Apnea: the Effect of Continuous Positive Airway Pressure." *NeuroImage*, Academic Press, 2 Nov. 2002,
    www.sciencedirect.com/science/article/pii/S1389945702001302

8. https://splitrockrehab.com/memory-improvement-seniors-sleep/

9. Guo, Shiyi et al. "Restless Legs Syndrome: From Pathophysiology to Clinical Diagnosis and Management" *Frontiers in aging neuroscience* vol. 9 171. 2 Jun. 2017, doi:10.3389/fnagi.2017.0017

10. Bogan, Richard K. "Effects of restless legs syndrome (RLS) on sleep" *Neuropsychiatric disease and treatment* vol. 2,4 (2006): 513-9.

11. "Serotonin and Sleep." *NeuroImage*, Academic Press, 13 June 2002, www.sciencedirect.com/science/article/pii/S1087079201901741.

12. https://www.healthline.com/health/dopamine-vs-serotonin

13. https://www.stanfordchildrens.org/en/topic/default?
id=newborn-sleep-patterns.

14. https://pharmacysolutionsonline.com/drug-induced-nutrient-depletion.php

15. Roux. "Restless Legs Syndrome: Impact on Sleep-Related Breathing Disorders." *Respirology. 2013 Feb; 18(2):238-45. Doi: 10.1111/J.1440-1843.2012.02249.x.*

16. Saaresranta, Tarja et al. "Sleep disordered breathing: is it different for females?" *ERJ open research* vol. 1,2 00063-2015. 3 Nov. 2015, doi:10.1183/23120541.00063-2015

17. Mathangi, D C et al. "Effect of REM sleep deprivation on the antioxidant status in the brain of Wistar rats" *Annals of neurosciences* vol. 19,4 (2012): 161-4.

18. Salin-Pascual, Rafael J., et al. "Differences in Sleep Variables, Blood Adenosine, and Body Temperature Between Hypothyroid and Euthyroid Rats Before and After REM Sleep Deprivation." *Sleep*, vol. 20, no. 11, 1997, pp. 957–962., doi:10.1093/sleep/20.11.957.

19. Matthew R. Cribbet, McKenzie Carlisle, Richard M. Cawthon, Bert N. Uchino, Paula G. Williams, Timothy W. Smith, Heather E. Gunn, Kathleen C. Light, Cellular Aging and Restorative Processes: Subjective Sleep Quality and Duration Moderate the Association between Age and Telomere Length in a Sample of Middle-Aged and Older Adults, *Sleep*, Volume 37, Issue 1, January 2014, Pages 65–70, https://doi.org/10.5665/sleep.3308

Chapter 4:

1. Costello, Rebecca B et al. "The effectiveness of melatonin for promoting healthy sleep: a rapid evidence assessment of the literature" *Nutrition journal* vol. 13 106. 7 Nov. 2014, doi:10.1186/1475-2891-13-106

2. Ferracioli-Oda, Eduardo et al. "Meta-analysis: melatonin for the treatment of primary sleep disorders" *PloS one* vol. 8,5 e63773. 17 May. 2013, doi:10.1371/journal.pone.0063773

3. Hinz, Marty et al. "5-HTP efficacy and contraindications" *Neuropsychiatric disease and treatment* vol. 8 (2012): 323-8.

4. 22. Gröber, Uwe and Klaus Kisters. "Influence of drugs on vitamin D and calcium metabolism" *Dermato-endocrinology* vol. 4,2 (2012): 158-66.

5. Rogers, Naomi L., and David F. Dinges. "Caffeine: Implications for Alertness in Athletes." *Clinics in Sports Medicine*, vol. 24, no. 2, 2005, doi:10.1016/j.csm.2004.12.012.

6. http://sleepeducation.org/news/2013/08/01/sleep-and-caffeine.

7. https://en.wikipedia.org/wiki/Mucuna_pruriens

8. Lampariello, Lucia Raffaella et al. "The Magic Velvet Bean of Mucuna pruriens" *Journal of traditional and complementary medicine* vol. 2,4 (2012): 331-9.

9. McCarthy, Cameron G et al. "A dietary supplement containing chlorophytum borivilianum and velvet bean improves sleep quality in men and women" *Integrative medicine insights* vol. 7 (2012): 7-14.

10. https://www.webmd.com/vitamins/ai/ingredientmono-104/california-poppy

11. Wankhede, Sachin et al. "Examining the effect of Withania somnifera supplementation on muscle strength and recovery: a randomized controlled trial" *Journal of the International Society of Sports Nutrition* vol. 12 43. 25 Nov. 2015, doi:10.1186/s12970-015-0104-9

12. Chandrasekhar, K et al. "A prospective, randomized double-blind, placebo-controlled study of safety and efficacy of a high-concentration full-spectrum extract of ashwagandha root in reducing stress and anxiety in adults" *Indian journal of psychological medicine* vol. 34,3 (2012): 255-62.

13. Sieradzan KA, Fox SH, Hill M, Dick JP, Crossman AR, Brotchie JM. Cannabinoids reduce levodopa-induced dyskinesia in Parkinson's disease: a pilot study.[Neurology. 2001]

14. https://cbdoilreview.org/cbd-cannabidiol/cbd-dosage/

15. Srivastava, Janmejai K et al. "Chamomile: A herbal medicine of the past with bright future" *Molecular medicine reports* vol. 3,6 (2010): 895-901.

16. Cohen, Marc Maurice. "Tulsi -Ocimum sanctum: A herb for all reasons" *Journal of Ayurveda and integrative medicine* vol. 5,4 (2014): 251-9.

17. Sharma MK, Kumar M, Kumar A. Ocimum sanctum aqueous leaf extract provides protection against mercury induced toxicity in Swiss albino mice. Indian J Exp Biol. 2002 Sep; 40(9):1079-82.

18. Talan, Jamie. "Lemon Balm May Boost the Brain / Researchers Focus on Memory Tests." *Newsday.com*, 4 Aug. 2003.

19. Newall CA, Anderson LA, Philpson JD. Herbal Medicine: A Guide for Healthcare Professionals. The Pharmaceutical Press; London: 1996.

20. M. I. Bianco, C. Lúquez**, L. I. T. de Jong, R. A. Fernández* Área Microbiolo. *Linden Flower (Tilia Spp.) as Potential Vehicle of Clostridium Botulinum Spores in the Transmission of Infant Botulism.*, doi:Rev. argent. microbiol. vol.41 no.4 Ciudad Autónoma de Buenos Aires Oct./Dec. 2009.

21. Rodriguez-Fragoso, Lourdes et al. "Risks and benefits of commonly used herbal medicines in Mexico" *Toxicology and applied pharmacology* vol. 227,1 (2007): 125-35.

22. Shikov, Alexander N., et al. "Effect of Leonurus Cardiaca Oil Extract in Patients with Arterial Hypertension Accompanied by Anxiety and Sleep Disorders." *Phytotherapy Research*, vol. 25, no. 4, 2010, pp. 540–543., doi:10.1002/ptr.3292.

23. Brock, Christine, et al. "American Skullcap (Scutellaria Lateriflora): A Randomised, Double-Blind Placebo-Controlled Crossover

Study of Its Effects on Mood in Healthy Volunteers." *Phytotherapy Research*, vol. 28, no. 5, 2013, pp. 692–698., doi:10.1002/ptr.5044.

24. Bent, Stephen et al. "Valerian for sleep: a systematic review and meta-analysis" *American journal of medicine* vol. 119,12 (2006): 1005-12.

25. Panossian, Alexander and Georg Wikman. "Effects of Adaptogens on the Central Nervous System and the Molecular Mechanisms Associated with Their Stress-Protective Activity" *Pharmaceuticals (Basel, Switzerland)* vol. 3,1 188-224. 19 Jan. 2010, doi:10.3390/ph3010188

26. Mao, Jun J et al. "Rhodiola rosea therapy for major depressive disorder: a study protocol for a randomized, double-blind, placebo-controlled trial" *Journal of clinical trials* vol. 4 (2014): 170.

27. Cicero, A.f.g., et al. "Effects Of Siberian Ginseng (Eleutherococcus Senticosus Maxim.) On Elderly Quality Of Life: A Randomized Clinical Trial." *Archives of Gerontology and Geriatrics*, vol. 38, 2004, pp. 69–73., doi:10.1016/j.archger.2004.04.012.

28. Zeng, Yawen et al. "Strategies of Functional Foods Promote Sleep in Human Being" *Current signal transduction therapy* vol. 9,3 (2014): 148-155.

29. Ajai KPandeyaAnumeghaGuptabMeenakshiTiwaribShilpaPrasadbAshutosh N.PandeybPramod K.YadavbAlkaSharmabKankshiSahubSyedAsrafuzzamancDoyil T.VengayilcTulsidas G.ShrivastavdShail KChaubeb. "Impact of Stress on Female Reproductive Health Disorders: Possible Beneficial Effects of Shatavari (Asparagus Racemosus)." doi:Biomedicine & Pharmacotherapy Volume 103, July 2018, Pages 46-49.

30. Park, J. Y., and K. H. Kim. "A Randomized, Double-Blind, Placebo-Controlled Trial of Schisandra Chinensis for Menopausal Symptoms." *Climacteric*, vol. 19, no. 6, 2016, pp. 574–580., doi:10.1080/13697137.2016.1238453.

31. https://www.sciencedirect.com/topics/medicine-and-dentistry/schisandra

32. Kripke, Daniel F. "Surprising view of insomnia and sleeping pills" *Sleep* vol. 36,8 1127-8. 1 Aug. 2013, doi:10.5665/sleep.2868

Chapter 5:

1. Lowry, Christopher A et al. "The Microbiota, Immunoregulation, and Mental Health: Implications for Public Health" *Current environmental health reports* vol. 3,3 (2016): 270-86.

2. *Metabolic Syndrome and Sleep Apnea -Ncbi.nlm.nih.gov.* www.ncbi.nlm.nih.gov/pmc/articles/PMC2464309/.

3. Gimeno, D et al. "Associations of C-reactive protein and interleukin-6 with cognitive symptoms of depression: 12-year follow-up of the Whitehall II study" *Psychological medicine* vol. 39,3 (2008): 413-23.

4. J Lipid Res. 1984 Dec 1;25(12):1277-94.

5. https://labtestsonline.org/tests/apo-b

6. Houston, Mark C. *What Your Doctor May Not Tell You about Heart Disease: the Revolutionary Book That Reveals the Truth behind Coronary Illnesses-and How You Can Fight Them.* Grand Central Life & Style, 2012.

7. JCI 2001: 108-399, AM J Clin Nutr 2010: 92:161

8. Houston, M.C. Handbook of Hypertension, Wiley Blackwell, Oxford, UK, 2009.

9. Houston, M.C. Vascular Biology in Clinical Practice. Hanley and Belfus, Philadelphia 2000.

10. Bryan, Nathan S., et al. "Oral Microbiome and Nitric Oxide: the Missing Link in the Management of Blood Pressure." *SpringerLink*, Springer, 28 Mar. 2017, link.springer.com/article/10.1007/s11906-017-0725-2.

11. Reddy, Y S et al. "Nitric oxide status in patients with chronic kidney disease" *Indian journal of nephrology* vol. 25,5 (2015): 287-91.
12. "A Stepwise Reduction in Plasma and Salivary Nitrite with Increasing Strengths of Mouthwash Following a Dietary Nitrate Load." *NeuroImage*, Academic Press, 15 Jan. 2016, www.sciencedirect.com/science/article/pii/S1089860316300027.
13. "Buteyko Method." *Wikipedia*, Wikimedia Foundation, 15 Feb. 2019, en.wikipedia.org/wiki/Buteyko_method.
14. Mann, Denise. "The Link Between Sleep and Diabetes." *WebMD*, WebMD, www.webmd.com/diabetes/features/diabetes-lack-of-sleep#1
15. www.Cdc.gov.
16. Diamant et al. Obesity Reviews, Volume 12: Issue 4 pages 272-281. April 2011
17. Lau WL, Kalantar-Zadach K. Vaziri ND. The Gut as a Source of Inflammation in Chronic Kidney Disease. Nephron 2015; 130:92-8.
18. Cani, Patrice D., et al. "Metabolic Endotoxemia Initiates Obesity and Insulin Resistance." *Diabetes*, American Diabetes Association, 1 July 2007, diabetes.diabetesjournals.org/content/56/7/1761.
19. *Sleep Disorders and Chronic Kidney Disease.* www.ncbi.nlm.nih.gov/pmc/articles/PMC4848147/.
20. "Impact of Sleep on Osteoporosis: Sleep Quality Is Associated with Bone Stiffness Index." *NeuroImage*, Academic Press, 29 Aug. 2016, www.sciencedirect.com/science/article/pii/S1389945716301423.
21. Larsen, J.P. & Tandberg, E. Mol Diag Ther (2001) 15: 267. https://doi.org/10.2165/00023210-200115040-00002.
22. Franzen, Peter L and Daniel J Buysse. "Sleep disturbances and depression: risk relationships for subsequent depression and therapeutic implications" *Dialogues in clinical neuroscience* vol. 10,4 (2008): 473-81.

23. Yong, Lee C., and Martin R. Peterson. "High Dietary Niacin Intake is Associated with Decreased Chromosome Translocation Frequency in Airline Pilots." British Journal of Nutrition, vol. 105, no. 04, 2010, pp. 496-505., doi:10.1017/s000711451000379x.

24. *Effects of Exercise on Sleep -Sportsmed.theclinics.com*. www.sportsmed. theclinics.com/article/S0278-5919(04)00139-5/pdf.

25. Beavers, Kristen M et al. "Effect of exercise training on chronic inflammation" *Clinica chimica acta; international journal of clinical chemistry* vol. 411,11-12 (2010): 785-93.

26. Woods, Jeffrey A et al. "Exercise, inflammation and aging" *Aging and disease*vol. 3,1 (2011): 130- 40.

27. "Sleep and Human Aging." *Scribd*, Scribd, www.scribd.com/ document/344386614/Sleep-and-Human-Aging.

28. Otte, Julie L et al. "Systematic review of sleep disorders in cancer patients: can the prevalence of sleep disorders be ascertained?" *Cancer medicine* vol. 4,2 (2014): 183-200.

29. Sateia, Michael J., and Bianca J. Lang. "Sleep and Cancer: Recent Developments." *Current Oncology Reports*, vol. 10, no. 4, 2008, pp. 309–318., doi:10.1007/s11912-008-0049-0.

30. Pessi T, Karhunen V, Karjalainen PP, Ylitalo A, Airaksinen JK, Niemi M, Pietila M, Lounatmaa K, Haapaniemi T, Lehtimaki T, Laaksonen R, Karhunen P, Mikkelsson J. Bacterial Signatures in Thrombus Aspirates of Patient with Myocardial Infarction. Circulation, 2013 Mar 19; 127(11): 1219-28, e1-6.

Chapter 6:

1. [Nutrition] Sites of Nutrient Absorption.png 262.68KB 2017-04-12 09:50:15

2. Holick MF. Vitamin D deficiency. N Engl J Med. 2007;357:266–81. doi: 10.1056/NEJMra070553. [PubMed] [CrossRef]

3. Holick MF, Chen TC. Vitamin D deficiency: a worldwide problem with health consequences. Am J Clin Nutr. 2008;87(suppl):1080S–6S.[PubMed]

4. Gao, Qi et al. "The Association between Vitamin D Deficiency and Sleep Disorders: A Systematic Review and Meta-Analysis" *Nutrients* vol. 10,10 1395. 1 Oct. 2018, doi:10.3390/nu10101395

5. Nair, R., Maseehm A. (2012). Vitamin D: The "sunshine" vitamin. Journal of Pharmacology & Pharmacotherapeutics. Apr-Jun; 3(2): 118-126. https://www.ncbi.nlm.nih.gov/pmc/articles/PMC3356951/

6. Office of Dietary Supplements. (2016). Vitamin D – Fact Sheet for Health Professionals. National Institutes of Health. https://ods.od.nih.gov/factsheets/VitaminD-HealthProfessional/

7. Vitamin D Food Source Chart, National Institutes of Health, 2009.

8. Okawa, et al. "Vitamin B 12 Treatment for Sleep-Wake Rhythm Disorders." *OUP Academic*, Oxford University Press, 1 Jan. 1990, academic.oup.com/sleep/article/13/1/15/2742708.

9. Ohta T, Ando K, Iwata T, Ozaki N, Kayukawa Y, Terashima M, Okada T, Kashara Y. Treatment of persistent sleep-wake schedule disorders in adolescents with methylcobalamin (vitamin B12) Sleep. 1991;14:414–18. [PubMed]

10. Sato-Mito N, Shibata S, Sasaki S, et al. Dietary intake is associated with human chronotype as assessed by both morningness–eveningness score and preferred midpoint of sleep in young Japanese women. Int J Food Sci. 2011;62:525–532.[PubMed]

11. Baldewicz, Teri, et al. "Plasma Pyridoxine Deficiency Is Related to Increased Psychological Distress in Recently Bereaved Homosexual Men." *Adolescence*, Libra Publishers Inc., 1 May 1998, miami.pure.elsevier.com/en/publications/plasma-pyridoxine-deficiency-is-related-to-increased-psychologica.

12. Ji, Xiaopeng, et al. "The Relationship between Micronutrient Status and Sleep Patterns: a Systematic Review." *Public Health Nutrition*, vol. 20, no. 04, 2016, pp. 687–701., doi:10.1017/s1368980016002603.

13. Schauss A, Costin C. Zinc as a nutrient in the treatment of eating disorders. Am J Nat Med. 1997 Dec;4: 8-10.

14. Bryce-Smith D, Simpson RI. Case of anorexia nervosa responding to zinc sulfate. Lancet. 1984 Aug11; 2(8398):350.

15. Bryce-Smith D, Simpson RI, Southon S, Johnson IT, Gee JM. Anorexia, depression, and zinc deficiency. Lancet. 1984 Nov17; 2(8412): 1162-1163

16. https://www.healthline.com/nutrition/iron-deficiency-signs-symptoms

17. https://www.webmd.com/diet/iron-rich-foods#1

18. https://www.healthline.com/nutrition/vitamin-b6-deficiency-symptoms#section6

19. https://www.webmd.com/diet/vitamin-b12-deficiency-symptoms-causes#1

20. McMaster University. "Science meets archaeology with discovery that dental X-rays reveal Vitamin D deficiency: Researchers find easy new method while looking for ways not to waste old teeth." ScienceDaily. ScienceDaily, 7 November 2017.

21. <www.sciencedaily.com/releases/2017/11/171107151311.htm>.

22. Gröber, Uwe and Klaus Kisters. "Influence of drugs on vitamin D and calcium metabolism" *Dermato-endocrinology* vol. 4,2 (2012): 158-66.

23. Magnesium and cardiovascular drugs: interactions and therapeutic role.Crippa G, Sverzellati E, Giorgi-Pierfranceschi M, Carrara GC.

24. Toh, James Wei Tatt, et al. "Hypomagnesaemia Associated with Long-Term Use of Proton Pump Inhibitors." *Gastroenterology*

Report, Oxford University Press, Aug. 2015, www.ncbi.nlm.nih.gov/pmc/articles/PMC4527261/.

25. https://pharmacysolutionsonline.com/drug-induced-nutrient-depletion.php

26. Riestra, Pia et al. "Circadian CLOCK gene polymorphisms in relation to sleep patterns and obesity in African Americans: findings from the Jackson heart study." *BMC genetics* vol. 18,1 58. 23 Jun. 2017, doi:10.1186/s12863-017-0522-6

27. Hu, Cheng, and Weiping Jia. "Linking MTNR1B Variants to Diabetes: The Role of Circadian Rhythms." *Diabetes 2016 Jun; 65(6): 1490-1492.*

28. Yager, James D. "Catechol-*O*-methyltransferase: characteristics, polymorphisms and role in breast cancer." *Drug discovery today. Disease mechanisms* vol. 9,1-2 (2012): e41-e46.

29. https://www.mayoclinic.org/drugs-supplements-same/art-20364924

Chapter 7:

1. Saaresranta, Tarja et al. "Sleep disordered breathing: is it different for females?" ERJ open research vol. 1,2 00063-2015. 3 Nov. 2015, doi:10.1183/23120541.00063-2015

2. Driver, Helen S., et al. "The Influence of the Menstrual Cycle on Upper Airway Resistance and Breathing During Sleep." Sleep, vol. 28, no. 4, 2005, pp. 449–456., doi:10.1093/sleep/28.4.449.

3. Helvaci, Nafiye et al. "Polycystic ovary syndrome and the risk of obstructive sleep apnea: a meta-analysis and review of the literature." Endocrine connections vol. 6,7 (2017): 437-445.

4. Saaresranta, Tarja et al. "Sleep disordered breathing: is it different for females?" ERJ open research vol. 1,2 00063-2015. 3 Nov. 2015, doi:10.1183/23120541.00063-2015

5. Wittert, Gary. "The relationship between sleep disorders and testosterone in men" Asian journal of andrology vol. 16,2 (2014): 262-5.

6. https://redcon1online.com/mucuna-pruriens/

7. Campos-Juanatey, Felix et al. "Effects of obstructive sleep apnea and its treatment over the erectile function: a systematic review" Asian journal of andrology vol. 19,3 (2016): 303-310.

8. "Thyroxine Replacement Therapy Reverses Sleep-Disordered Breathing in Patients with Primary Hypothyroidism." Sleep Medicine, Elsevier, 28 Sept. 2005, www.sciencedirect.com/science/article/pii/S1389945705001103.

9. Winkelman JW1, Goldman H, Piscatelli N, Lukas SE, Dorsey CM, Cunningham S. Are Thyroid Function Tests Necessary in Patients with Suspected Sleep Apnea?. Sleep. 1996 Dec;19(10):790-3.

10. Sridhar, G R et al. "Sleep in thyrotoxicosis." Indian journal of endocrinology and metabolism vol. 15,1 (2011): 23-6. doi:10.4103/2230-8210.77578

11. Chien-Hsiang Weng, Yi-Huei Chen, and Tseng-Hsi Lin Xun Luo. "Thyroid Disorders and Breast Cancer Risk in Asian Population: a Nationwide Population-Based Case–Control Study in Taiwan." BMJ Open, British Medical Journal Publishing Group, 1 Mar. 2018, bmjopen.bmj.com/content/8/3/e020194.

12. Breast Cancer in Association with Thyroid Disorders www.ncbi.nlm.nih.gov/pmc/articles/PMC314421/.

13. Dudhia, Sonal B and Bhavin B Dudhia. "Undetected hypothyroidism: A rare dental diagnosis" Journal of oral and maxillofacial pathology : JOMFP vol. 18,2 (2014): 315-9.

14. Chrousos G, Vgontzas AN, Kritikou I. HPA Axis and Sleep. [Updated 2016 Jan 18]. In: Feingold KR, Anawalt B, Boyce A, et al., editors. Endotext [internet]. South Dartmouth (MA): MDText.com, Inc.; 2000-. Available from: https://www.ncbi.nlm.nih.gov/books/NBK279071/

15. Michelson D, Galliven E, Hill L, et al. Chronic imipramine is associated with diminished hypothalamic-pituitary-adrenal axis responsivity in healthy humans. J Clin Endocrinol Metab 1997;82:2601-2606

16. Rodenbeck A, Cohrs S, Jordan W, et al. The sleep-improving effects of doxepin are paralleled by a normalized plasma cortisol secretion in primary insomnia. A placebo-controlled, double-blind, randomized, cross-over study followed by an open treatment over 3 weeks. Psychopharmacology (Berl) 2003;170:423-428

17. Vgontzas AN, Zoumakis E, Bixler EO, et al. Selective effects of CPAP on sleep apnoea-associated manifestations. Eur J Clin Invest 2008;38:585-595

18. Vgontzas AN, Pejovic S, Zoumakis E, et al. Hypothalamic-pituitary-adrenal axis activity in obese men with and without sleep apnea: effects of continuous positive airway pressure therapy. J Clin Endocrinol Metab 2007;92:4199-4207

19. Gillin JC, Jacobs LS, Fram DH, Snyder F. Acute effect of a glucocorticoid on normal human sleep. Nature 1972;237:398-399

20. Shipley JE, Schteingart DE, Tandon R, Starkman MN. Sleep architecture and sleep apnea in patients with Cushing disease. Sleep 1992;15:514-518

21. Moldofsky H, Lue FA, Eisen J, Keystone E, Gorczynski RM. The relationship of interleukin-1 and immune functions to sleep in humans. Psychosom Med 1986;48:309-318

22. Fernandez-Real JM, Vayreda M, Richart C, et al. Circulating interleukin 6 levels, blood pressure, and insulin sensitivity in apparently healthy men and women. J Clin Endocrinol Metab 2001;86:1154-1159

23. Shoham S, Davenne D, Cady AB, Dinarello CA, Krueger JM. Recombinant tumor necrosis factor and interleukin 1 enhance slow-wave sleep. Am J Physiol 1987;253:R142-149

24. Kapas L, Krueger JM. Tumor necrosis factor-beta induces sleep, fever, and anorexia. Am J Physiol 1992;263:R703-707

25. Floyd RA, Krueger JM. Diurnal variation of TNF alpha in the rat brain. Neuroreport 1997;8:915-918

26. Papanicolaou DA, Wilder RL, Manolagas SC, Chrousos GP. The pathophysiologic roles of interleukin-6 in human disease. Ann Intern Med 1998;128:127-137

27. https://en.wikipedia.org/wiki/Cushing%27s_syndrome

28. Shoham S, Davenne D, Cady AB, Dinarello CA, Krueger JM. Recombinant tumor necrosis factor and interleukin 1 enhance slow-wave sleep. Am J Physiol 1987;253:R142-149

29. Kapas L, Krueger JM. Tumor necrosis factor-beta induces sleep, fever, and anorexia. Am J Physiol 1992;263:R703-707

30. Floyd RA, Krueger JM. Diurnal variation of TNF alpha in the rat brain. Neuroreport 1997;8:915-918

31. https://www.mayoclinic.org/diseases-conditions/addisons-disease/symptoms-causes/syc-20350293

32. https://en.wikipedia.org/wiki/Cushing%27s_syndrome

Chapter 8:

1. Relationship of Childhood Abuse and Household Dysfunction to Many of the Leading Causes of Death in Adults. Felitti, Vincent J et al. American Journal of Preventive Medicine, Volume 14, Issue 4, 245 -258

2 Chapman, DP, et al. "Adverse Childhood Experiences and Sleep Disturbances in Adults." *Sleep Medicine*, Elsevier, 24 June 2011, www.sciencedirect.com/science/article/pii/S1389945711001663.

3 Schneiderman, Janet U., et al. "Longitudinal Relationship Between Mental Health Symptoms and Sleep Disturbances and Duration in Maltreated and Comparison Adolescents." *Journal of Ado-*

lescent Health, vol. 63, no. 1, 2018, pp. 74–80., doi:10.1016/j. jadohealth.2018.01.011.

4   Human sleep in 60 Hz magnetic fields.[Bioelectromagnetics. 1999]

5.   Associations of frequent sleep insufficiency with health-related quality of life and health behaviors.[Sleep Med. 2005]

6.   Barsam, Tayebeh, et al. "Effect of Extremely Low Frequency Electromagnetic Field Exposure on Sleep Quality in High Voltage Substations." *Iranian Journal of Environmental Health Science & Engineering*, vol. 9, no. 1, 2012, p. 15., doi:10.1186/1735-2746-9-15.

7.   Röösli M, Moser M, Baldinini Y, Meier M, Braun-Fahrländer C. Symptoms of ill health ascribed to electromagnetic field exposure–a questionnaire survey. Int J Hyg Environ Health. 2004;207(2):141–50. doi: 10.1078/1438-4639-00269.[PubMed] [CrossRef]

8.   Department of Pain Medicine, Palliative Care and Integrative Medicine. *Pediatric Integrative Medicine Reference Card*. Children's Minnesota., Mar. 2017.

9.   Church, Dawson, and David Feinstein. "The Manual Stimulation of Acupuncture Points in the Treatment of Post-Traumatic Stress Disorder: A Review of Clinical Emotional Freedom Techniques." *Medical acupuncture* vol. 29,4 (2017): 194-205. doi:10.1089/ acu.2017.1213

Chapter 9:

1.   Röösli, Christof, et al. "Long-Term Results and Complications Following Uvulopalatopharyngoplasty in 116 Consecutive Patients." European Archives of Oto-Rhino-Laryngology, vol. 263, no. 8, 2006, pp. 754–758., doi:10.1007/s00405-006-0051-9.

2.   *CASE REPORT: NightLase Procedure Laser Snoring and Sleep* …www.laserandhealthacademy.com/media/objave/academy/ priponke/sippus_laha_2015_onlinefirst.pdf.

3. https://www.respshop.com/resource/history-of-cpap/
4. Pinto VL, Sharma S. Continuous Positive Airway Pressure (CPAP) [Updated 2019 Jan 20]. In: StatPearls [internet]. Treasure Island (FL): StatPearls Publishing; 2019 Jan-. Available from: https://www.ncbi.nlm.nih.gov/books/NBK482178/
5. Aarab, Ghizlane, et al. "Oral Appliance Therapy versus Nasal Continuous Positive Airway Pressure in Obstructive Sleep Apnea: a Randomized, Placebo-Controlled Trial on Psychological Distress." SpringerLink, Springer Berlin Heidelberg, 12 Jan. 2017, link. springer.com/article/10.1007/s00784-016-2045-3.
6. Lam, B, et al. "Craniofacial Profile in Asian and White Subjects with Obstructive Sleep Apnoea." Thorax, BMJ Group, June 2005, www.ncbi.nlm.nih.gov/pmc/articles/PMC1747424/.
7. ALF brochure from Angie Tenholder, DDS
8. https://en.wikipedia.org/wiki/Mallampati_score
9. NON-SURGICAL, UPPER AIRWAY REMODELING FOR OBSTRUCTIVE...daks2k3a4ib2z.cloudfront.net/59419022ff1d-4150cb0158a6/5947f1b0e797e633076f22fa_1.pdf.
10. Dds, M Cortes, and Me Wallace-Nadolski. "0636 Non-Surgical, Upper Airway Remodeling For Uars." Sleep, vol. 40, no. suppl_1, 2017, doi:10.1093/sleepj/zsx050.635.
11. G, Felix Liao Dave Singh. "Resolution of Sleep Bruxism Using Biomimetic Oral Appliance Therapy: A Case Report." Journal of Sleep Disorders & Therapy, vol. 04, no. 04, 2015, doi:10.4172/2167-0277.1000204.
12. Singh, Dave. "Resolution of Pediatric Chronic Rhinitis Using Biomimetic Oral Appliance Therapy: A Case Report." Open Journal of Clinical and Medical Case Reports, Volume 2, no. Issue 4, 2016, pp. 1–6.

Chapter 10:

1. "Clinical Psychology of Oral Health: The Link Between Teeth and Emotions." *SAGE Journals*, journals.sagepub.com/doi/full/10.1177/2158244017728319.

2. Nuttall, N. M., Steele, J. G., Pine, C. M., White, D., & Pitts, N. B. (2001). Adult dental health survey: The impact of oral health on people in the UK in 1998. *British Dental Journal, 190*, 121-126

3. Valenti VE, Guida HL, Vanderlei LC, Rogue AL, Ferreira C, Silva TD, Manhabusque KV, Fuijimori M, Abreu LC: Relationship between cadiac autonomicregulation and auditory mechanisms: importance for growth and development. J Hum Growth Dev 2013, 2013:23.*Effects of Orofacial Myofunctional Therapy on…* aomtinfo.org/wp-content/uploads/2015/03/effects-of-orofacial-my-ofunctional-therapy-on-temporomandibular-disorders.pdf.

4. Hamer, Dr. med. Mag. Theol. Ryke Geerd. "Scientific Chart of Germanic New Medicine. ". Amici di Dirk, Eidciones de la Nueva Medicina, S.L. , December 2007; page 13-14.

5. Sympathetic and Parasympathetic Nervous Systems. www.istockphoto.com

6. *Effects of Orofacial Myofunctional Therapy on…* aomtinfo.org/wp-content/uploads/2015/03/effects-of-orofacial-myofunction-al-therapy-on-temporomandibular-disorders.pdf.

7. Camacho, Macario, et al. "Myofunctional Therapy to Treat Obstructive Sleep Apnea: A Systematic Review and Meta-Analysis." *Sleep*, Associated Professional Sleep Societies, LLC, 1 May 2015, www.ncbi.nlm.nih.gov/pubmed/25348130.

8. Saper RB, Lemaster C, Yoga, Physical Therapy, or Education for Chronic Low Back Pain: A Randomized Noninferiority Trial. Ann Intern Med. 2017 Jul 18; 167 (2): 85-94.

9. de Felício, Cláudia Maria et al. "Obstructive sleep apnea: focus on myofunctional therapy." *Nature and science of sleep* vol. 10 271-286. 6 Sep. 2018, doi:10.2147/NSS. S141132

10. *Sleep Alterations Following Exposure to Stress Predict...*www.ncbi.nlm.nih.gov/pmc/articles/PMC4827610/.

11. Choi, Inho, et al. "The New Era of the Lymphatic System: No Longer Secondary to the Blood Vascular System." *Cold Spring Harbor Perspectives in Medicine*, Cold Spring Harbor Laboratory Press, Apr. 2012, www.ncbi.nlm.nih.gov/pmc/articles/ PMC3312397/.

12. Burns, Sylvia L. "Concussion Treatment Using Massage Techniques: a Case Study." *International journal of therapeutic massage & bodywork* vol. 8,2 12-7. 9 Jun. 2015

13. Hsiao, Pei-Chi et al. "Risk of breast cancer recurrence in patients receiving manual lymphatic drainage: a hospital-based cohort study." *Therapeutics and clinical risk management* vol. 11 349-58. 27 Feb. 2015, doi:10.2147/TCRM. S79118.

14. Wetzler, Gail et al. "CranioSacral Therapy and Visceral Manipulation: A New Treatment Intervention for Concussion Recovery." *Medical acupuncture* vol. 29,4 (2017): 239-248. doi:10.1089/ acu.2017.1222.

15. Bourke, Mary and Cole Clayton. *Myo Munchee: A Practitioner User Guide.* Vol. 1. The Junction NSW: Myo Munchee Australia, 2018.

About the Author

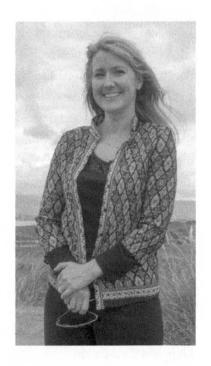

Amy M. Dayries, D.M.D. has practiced general dentistry in Roswell (near where she grew up) since 1996 after graduating from the Medical College of Georgia School of Dentistry and having attended Emory University (majoring in Chemistry) for her undergraduate work. Dr. Dayries is passionate about smile design, health, and nutrition, and she prefers to take a natural, holistic, or biologic (integrative) approach to care when possible. Patient health and satisfaction are her ultimate goals. Dr. Dayries has focused her family practice on dental function and aesthetics such as bonding and veneers for years, but she also developed an appreciation that elements and compounds compatible for one patient may aggravate sensitivities or allergies in another patient. She realizes that appreciating and educating about the overall health of her patients is a large part of helping a patient obtain their most radiant, aesthetic smile.

Her own personal experiences with lead and mercury toxicity and as a mother and Girl Scout Leader sparked Dr. Dayries' passion for nutritional counseling and the herbal arts. Dr. Dayries often recommends lifestyle choices as part of a regimen to improve oral and systemic health to patients.

Dr. Dayries' Extra Dental Education and Current Professional **Affiliations/Activities**:

National Spokesman and Educator for the American Dental Association on Integrative Health and Holistic Dental topics. Has lectured at the 2017 and 2018 American Dental Association's National Convention and for other healthcare audiences around the United States.

Whole Healing Radio Show with Dr. Amy Dayries, featured with the United Intentions Network. Podcasts available on either FaceBook page for Amy Dayries-Ling, on www.UnitedIntentionsMedia.org or YouTube "Amy Dayries." Live broadcasts can be heard on Atlanta's FM 99.1 on alternating Thursday evenings at 6 pm.

Fellow, Academy of Integrative Health and Medicine. First dentist to graduate from this two-year inter-professional program for healthcare providers.

Studied herbal medicine under the guidance of notable author, clinician and teacher Dr. Tieraona Low Dog, M.D.

Dr. Dayries resides in Roswell, Georgia with her husband, Mike Ling, and their children. Over the years, Dr. Dayries has enjoyed teaching Sunday School, being a Girl Scout leader, jogging, and gardening.

Dr. Dayries also does healthy lifestyle seminars at local farmers markets and has written for some local publications in the Atlanta area.

Dr. Dayries can be contacted at (770) 753-0067 or at www.Whole-HealingDental.com.